£40

Mental Disorders and Cognitive Deficits in Multiple Sclerosis

Editors

*K. Jensen, *L. Knudsen, *E. Stenager and I Grant

Clinical Neuropsychiatric Research Unit, Odense University Hospital, Denmark

Medical Center & Department of Psychiatry, University of California School of Medicine, San Diego, U.S.A.

The cover illustration courtesy of Finn Hjernöe, Denmark

MENTAL DISORDERS AND COGNITIVE DEFICITS IN MULTIPLE SCLEROSIS

Edited by

K. JENSEN, L. KNUDSEN, E. STENAGER AND I. GRANT

John Libbey
LONDON · PARIS

British Library Cataloguing in Publication Data

Mental disorders.
1. Man. Multiple sclerosis. Neurological aspects
I. Grant, I. II. Jensen, P. K. III. Series
616.8'34

ISBN 0-86196-180-3

First published in 1989 by

John Libbey & Company Ltd
13 Smith's Yard, Summerley St., London SW18 4HR, UK. (01) 497 2777

John Libbey Eurotext Ltd
6 rue Blanche, 92120 Montrouge, France. (1) 47 35 85 52

Phototypeset by Dobbie Typesetting Limited, Plymouth, Devon.
Printed in Great Britain by Whitstable Litho Ltd, Whitstable, Kent.

CONTENTS

PREFACE

In earlier research not much attention was paid to the mental disorders often seen in conjunction with multiple sclerosis. This is surprising, considering the disease gives rise to widespread lesions in the central nervous system so that impairment of intellectual function and other mental disorders may be expected.

While working in this field we found that only few research centres in the world engage in research on this aspect of multiple sclerosis. We therefore decided to organize a symposium to further an exchange of ideas and experiences among the few researchers working in this area. The title chosen for the symposium was: Mental Disorders, Cognitive Defects and their Treatment in Multiple Sclerosis.

The symposium took place on November 18–21, 1987, in Odense, Denmark. Our initiative was greeted with great interest by all the scientific centres approached, most of which were represented at our symposium.

Realizing that this symposium was the first of its kind to be held on an international level and that papers presented therefore would be of fundamental value for research on multiple sclerosis, we decided to combine the presentations in a publication in the hope that the book would be of inspiration to others.

We know from our work with patients suffering from multiple sclerosis that it is of utmost importance to be aware of the psychic resources of the individual patient when planning a future that allows for a varying degree of handicap. Too often patients are forced into education or employment situations that contain the risk of frustration and failure when intellectual capacity proves to be insufficient. We are therefore convinced that a publication of this kind will be useful for physicians and psychologists in their efforts to build up a future with the highest quality attainable for our patients.

We feel that the deep interest shown in our symposium clearly illustrates the need for greater endeavour in our work and it is our hope that this book will enable researchers to continue theirs, though with greater awareness of the psychiatric and psychological features the disease presents.

The symposium and publication of the book have been made possible by the generous support received from the Danish Multiple Sclerosis Society, the National Multiple Sclerosis Society, U. S. A., l'Association pour la Recherche sur la Sclérose en Plaques, France, and the World Federation for Mental Health. In addition, support was received from a number of Danish Foundations: Fonden for Scleroseramte på Fyn, ingeniør K. A. Rohde og hustrus legat, Smith & Co.'s Fond, and Bikubenfonden. We wish to express our deep appreciation to all these sources.

We should also like to thank Shiela Hauge and Dorinda Schnack for their help both when organizing the symposium and during it. We should like to thank Shiela Hauge in addition for help in arranging the manuscripts for publication.

Odense
and
La Jolla
1989

Knud Jensen
Lone Knudsen
Egon Stenager
Igor Grant

1

HISTORICAL NOTES ON MENTAL ASPECTS OF MULTIPLE SCLEROSIS

Egon Stenager, Lone Knudsen, and Knud Jensen

Clinical Neuropsychiatric Research Unit, Departments of Neurology, Clinical Psychology and Psychiatry, Odense University Hospital, Odense, Denmark

> 'There is a marked enfeeblement of the memory; conceptions are formed slowly; the intellectual and emotional faculties are blunted in their totality. The dominant feeling in the patients appears to be a sort of almost stupid indifference in reference to all things. It is not rare to see them give way to foolish laughter for no cause and sometimes melt into tears without reason. Nor is it rare amidst the state of mental depression to find psychic disorders arise which assume one or the other of the classic forms of mental alienation.'
>
> J. M. Charcot (1825–1893)[1]

Charcot's epoch-making description not only of the neurological but also of the mental symptoms of multiple sclerosis (MS) became the norm for the conception of the psyche of patients suffering from that disease. Through Charcot's famous Tuesday lectures and lecture notes, knowledge of MS spread and for a long period most investigations of the disease agreed with his description. In their publications, his contemporaries Vulpian (1826–1887)[2] and Gowers (1845–1915)[3] also comment on mental symptoms, although Gowers pointed out that they were seldom severe. Even before Charcot's significant book appeared in 1872, a number of descriptions of mental symptoms seen in MS patients were made.

Early descriptions

Pratt[4] reports that the first description of mental symptoms seen in connection with MS are mentioned in the diary of Augustus d'Este (1774–1848). In 1833 a Danish medical journal[5] referred to a short article describing memory problems entitled 'Peculiar, Ordinary Paralysis'. A few years later, in 1838, an important event in medical literature occurred when the disease entity now known as multiple sclerosis was given a patho-anatomical description by Carswell[6] (1783–1853). Carswell worked in a Paris hospital for a period, where he seems to have collaborated with a French colleague, J. Cruveillier (1835–1842), who wrote Atlas d'Anatomie Pathologique[7] in which for the first time, clinical symptoms were related to patho-anatomical findings. A few years later, Frerichs[8] (1819–1885) also noted mental symptoms in the form of intellectual impairment in two of four cases, and in 1856 his pupil, Valentiner[9] described two cases with mental symptoms in the form of denial, overestimation of self and melancholy. From these early descriptions of MS, it became clear that cognitive and mental changes were features of the disease.

First systematic investigations

In 1897, after Charcot's death, Buzzard[10] described nine cases of MS which were mistakenly diagnosed as hysteria, but apart from that, more than 10 years passed before new reports appeared. However, early in the 20th century several descriptions were published, first in the form of case reports[11–18] which noted a variety of mental symptoms. During the same period, knowledge of this aspect of the disease spread from France to Germany, and later to the United States. According to early publications there, the disease was considered rare,[14] but in 1922 Wechsler[19] acknowledged that it was a common disease and that it was often accompanied by mental symptoms.

The many case reports published since have led to more systematic investigations being carried out in psychiatric departments[20,21] and these have shown, in contrast to those carried out in neurological departments,[22,23] that many patients suffer from mental disorders. No particular attention was paid to selection criteria, which varied and were often lacking, and there was therefore disagreement on the frequency of the mental symptoms[24,25] and also on whether they were specific for MS.[25,26]

As in the studies of Charcot, the investigations were clinical assessments and therefore covered an evaluation of cognitive and mental symptoms. An important publication from the period is the thesis of A. Ombredane,[23] Paris 1929, which underlined the mental symptoms of the disease.

Transition period 1930–1950

In the early 1930s there was great investigational activity in the field, but in the succeeding years only few studies were carried out.[20,27–32] However, significant progress was made. The first investigation using reproducible selection criteria and covering consecutive admissions to a neurological department was made,[27] and others appeared focusing on specific mental disorders, e.g. psychoses,[28,29] and behavioural disturbances.[30] Longworthy[31,32–33] even advised treatment of mental disorders in patients with MS.

Developments after the 1950s

With a few exceptions, attention up to this time had focused on both cognitive and mental disorders. Furthermore, and again with a few exceptions,[34,35] with the development of improved techniques in neuropsychology the overall evaluation of cerebral functioning in MS patients was discontinued. Investigations now dealt exclusively with either neuropsychological or psychiatric aspects.

Neuropsychological investigations

In the past 35 years numerous neuropsychological investigations have been performed on MS patients.[26–66] These investigations are difficult to compare, partly due to their adherence to different neuropsychological schools and partly because of the absence of any epidemiological consideration in the selection of patients. In recent years studies have dealt with memory function,[56–59] methodology,[62–63] and some have contained comparisons with other diseases,[37,65,66] for example muscular dystrophy. For many years questionnaires concerning personality characteristics have also been used.[67–73]

Even in the neuropsychological studies there has been a tendency to focus exclusively on memory function and on the use of new techniques which reveal greater detail.[57,58]

Psychiatric investigations

In psychiatric investigations from the 1950s,[74–80] 1960s,[81–84] 1970s,[85–87] and in the 1980s,[88–91] there has been a revival in the case report form. These case report publications are in many respects comparable with those from the start of this century.

During the same period, comprehensive investigations have appeared,[35,92–94] in one of which the Rorschach test was even applied.[94] But as in the neuropsychological investigations, a tendency towards exclusivism is again seen, in that some studies focused entirely on mental traumas connected with onset of MS,[95–98] while others have concentrated on depressive symptoms alone[99–103] or on behavioural disturbances.[104,105] Furthermore, using new techniques, attempts were made to explain the mental symptoms through localization of the lesions in the brain.[106,107]

Conclusion

In the past 150 years, investigation of mental disorders in MS has developed from broad, descriptive studies to very detailed investigations. The majority of the investigations have disregarded the importance of epidemiological selection criteria and methodology. Consequently they are difficult to compare.

It is therefore necessary for further investigations on mental disorders and cognitive deficits to be carried out using representative, epidemiological selection criteria, and for the methods used to be described clearly so that we can gain a deeper understanding of the mental symptoms seen in multiple sclerosis.

References

1 Charcot, J. M. (1872): *Leçons sur la maladies du system nerveux faits a la salpatriére.* 2nd. edn. Paris: Tomé.

2 Vulpian, A. (1886): *Maladies du systéme nerveux.* Paris: Doin.

3 Gowers, W. R. (1888): *A manual of diseases of the nervous system.* Vol. 2. London: Churchill.

4 Pratt, R. T. C. (1951): An investigation of the psychiatric aspects of disseminated sclerosis. *J. Neurol. Neurosurg. Psychiatry* **14**, 326–335.

5 Anonymous (1833): Mærkelig, almindelig lamhed. *Bibliotek for Læger* **18**, 192–193.

6 Carswell, R. (1838): *Pathological anatomy. Illustrations of the elementary forms of disease.* London.

7 Cruveillier, J. (1835–1842): *Atlas d'anatomie pathologique.* Livraison XXXII et XXXVII. Paris.

8 Frerichs, F. T. (1849): Ueber Hirnsklerose. *Archiv für die Gesamte Medizin* **10**, 334–350.

9 Valentiner, W. (1856): Über die Sclerose des Gehirns und Rückenmarks. *Deutsche Klinik* **14**, 147–151.

10 Buzzard, T. (1897): Insular sclerosis and hysteria. *Lancet* **i**, 1–4.

11 Lannois, M. (1903): Troubles psychiques dans un cas de sclérose en plaques. *Rev. Neurol.* **11**, 876–881.
12 Mönkemöller (1922): Multiple Sklerose und Geisteskrankheit. *Archiv für Psychiatrie* **66**, 459–528.
13 Christiansen, V. (1901): Tilfælde af disseminerede lidelser i centralnervesystemet. *Bibliotek for Læger* **96**, 330–364.
14 Spiller, W. G. & Camp, C. D. (1904): Multiple sclerosis, with a report of two additional cases. *J. Nerv. Ment. Dis.* **31**, 433–445.
15 Dercum, F. X. (1912): A case of multiple cerebral sclerosis, presenting unusual symptoms suggesting paresis. *J. A. M. A.* **59**, 1612–1613.
16 Ross, M. (1915): The mental symptoms in disseminated sclerosis. *Rev. Neurol. Psychiatry* **13**, 361–373.
17 Brown, S. & Davis, T. K. (1922): The mental symptoms of multiple sclerosis. *Arch. Neurol. Psychiatry* **7**, 629–634.
18 Howes, S. F. H. (1927): Psychosis with multiple sclerosis. *Boston Medical and Surgical Journal* **196**, 310–315.
19 Wechsler, I. S. (1922): Statistics of multiple sclerosis. *Brain* **8**, 59–75.
20 Saethre, H. (1932): Psychische Störungen bei Multiple Sklerose. *Acta Psyk. et Neurol.* **7**, 511–543.
21 Moser, K. (1924): Zur Bedeutung Psychischer Störungen in Multiple Sclerose. *Archiv für Psychiatrie und Nervenkrankheit* **71**, 694–700.
22 Sachs, B. & Friedman, E. D. (1922): General symptomatology and differential diagnoses of disseminated sclerosis. *Arch. Neurol. Psychiatry* **7**, 551–560.
23 Ombredane, A. (1929): *Sur les troubles mentaux de la sclérose en plaques*. Thesis. Paris: Les Presses Universitaires de France.
24 Runge, W. (1928): *Bunke's handbuch der geisteskrankheiten*. Siebenter Bind, pp. 616–630. Spezieller Teil III: Springer, Berlin.
25 Guillain, G. (1924): Rapport sur la sclérose en plaque. *Rev. Neurol.* **1**, 648–683.
26 Cottrell, S. S. & Wilson, S. A. K. (1926): The affective symptomatology of disseminated sclerosis. *J. Neurol. Psychopathol.* **7**, 1–30.
27 Borberg, N. C. & Zahle, V. (1946): On the psychopathology of disseminated sclerosis. *Acta Psychol. et Neurol.* **21**: 75–89.
28 Arbuse, D. I. (1938); Psychotic manifestations in disseminated sclerosis. *J. Mount Sinai Hospital.* Nov./Dec.: 403–410.
29 Malone, W. H. (1937): Psychosis with multiple sclerosis. *Medical Bulletin of the Veterans Administration* **14**, 113–117.
30 Sugar, C. & Nadell, R. (1943): Mental symptoms in multiple sclerosis. *J. Nerv. Ment. Dis.* **98**, 267–280.
31 Langworthy, O. R., Kolb, L. C. & Androp, S. (1941): Disturbances of behaviour in patients with disseminated sclerosis. *Am. J. Psychiatry* **28**, 243–249.
32 Langworthy, O. R. (1948): Relation of personality problems to onset and progress of multiple sclerosis. *Arch. Neurol. Psychiatry* **59**, 13–28.
33 Langworthy, O. R. (1950): A survey of the maladjustment problems in multiple sclerosis and the possibility of psychotherapy. *Proc. Assoc. Res. Nerv. Ment. Dis.* **28**, 598–611.
34 Steller, U. & Bech, U. (1987): Durchgangssyndrom als Frühsymptom einer Multiplen Sklerose. *Nervenarzt* **58**, 256–260.
35 Bender, I. (1950): Die Psychichen Veränderungen bei der Multiplen Sklerose. *Deutsche Zeitschrift Zur Nervenheilkunden* **163**, 483–526.
36 Heaton, R. K., Nelson, L. M., Thompson, D. S., Burks, J. S. & Franklin, A. M. (1985): Neuropsychological findings in relapsing-remitting and chronic progressive multiple sclerosis. *J. Consult. Clin. Psychol.* **53**, 103–110.
37 Jambor, K. L. (1969): Cognitive functioning in multiple sclerosis. *Br. J. Psychiatry* **115**, 765–775.
38 Matthews, C. G., Cleeland, C. S., Hopper, C. L. (1970): Neuropsychological patterns in multiple sclerosis. *Dis. Nerv. System* **31**, 161–170.
39 Reitan, R. M., Reed, J. C. & Dyken, M. L. (1971): Cognitive, psychomotor and motor correlates of multiple sclerosis. *J. Nerv. Ment. Dis.* **153**, 218–224.
40 Goldstein, G. & Shelley, C. H. (1974): Neuropsychological diagnosis of multiple sclerosis in a neuropsychiatric setting. *J. Nerv. Ment. Dis.* **158**, 280–290.

41 Ivnik, R. J. (1978): Neuropsychological performance as a function of the duration of MS-related symptomatology. *J. Clin. Psychol.* **46**, 304–312.
42 Ivnik, R. J. (1978): Neuropsychological stability in multiple sclerosis. *J. Consult. Psychol.* **46**, 913–923.
43 Marsh, G. G. (1980): Disability and intellectual function in multiple sclerosis patients. *J. Nerv. Ment. Dis.* **168**, 758–762.
44 Staples, D. & Lincoln, N. B. (1979): Intellectual impairment in multiple sclerosis and its relation to functional abilities. *Rheumatol. Rehabil.* **18**, 153–160.
45 Motte, J. F., Violet, L. & Derceux, J. F. (1982): Deterioration mentale et sclérose en plaques. *LARC Medical,* 88–9.
46 Peyser, J. M., Edwards, K. R., Poser, C. M. & Filskov, S. B. (1980): Cognitive function in patients with multiple sclerosis. *Arch. Neurol.* **37**, 577–579.
47 Medaer, R., De Smedt L., Swerts, M. & Geutjens, J. (1984): Use of rating scales to reflect cognitive and mental functioning in multiple sclerosis. *Acta Neurol. Scand.* **101**, 65–67.
48 Lanarés, J., Assal, G. & Regli, F. (1984): Etude neuropsycholoque clinique d'une population de patients atteints de sclérose en plaque. *Schweiz. Med. Wochenschr.* **114**, 141–144.
49 Diers, W. C. & Brown, C. C. (1950): Psychometric patterns associated with multiple sclerosis. *Arch. Neurol. Psychiatry* **63**, 760–765.
50 Gilberstadt, H. & Farkas, E. (1961): Another look at MMPI profile types in multiple sclerosis. *J. Consult. Psychol.* **25**, 440–444.
51 Hirchenfang, S. & Benton, J. (1966): Note on intellectual changes in multiple sclerosis. *Percept. Motor Skills* **22**, 786.
52 Javal, I. (1959): Etude psychometrique d'un groupe de sujets atteints de sclérose en plaques. *Schweiz Zeitschr. für psychologie und ihre Anwendungen* **18**, 299–302.
53 Sonkin, N. & Tomkin, A. (1963): Intellectual impairment in multiple sclerosis. *Ir. Med. J.* **46**, 262–265.
54 Young, A. C., Saunders, J. & Ponsford, J. R. (1976): Mental change as an early feature of multiple sclerosis. *J. Neurol. Neurosurg. Psychiatry* **39**, 1008–1013.
55 Fink, S. L. & Houser, H. B. (1966): An investigation of physical and intellectual changes in multiple sclerosis. *Arch. Phys. Rehabil.* **47**, 52–61.
56 Parsons, O. A., Kenneth, D. S. & Arenberg, D. (1957): Impairment of abstractivity ability in multiple sclerosis. *J. Nerv. Ment. Dis.* **125**, 221–225.
57 Rao, S. M., Glatt, S., Hammeke, T. A. *et al.* (1985): Chronic progressive multiple sclerosis. *Arch. Neurol.* **42**, 678–682.
58 Rao, S. M., Hammeke, T. A., McQuillen, M. P., Khatri, B. O. & Lloyd, D. (1984): Memory disturbances in chronic multiple sclerosis. *Arch. Neurol.* **41**, 625–631.
59 Beatty, P. A. & Gange, J. J. (1977): Neuropsychological aspects of multiple sclerosis. *J. Nerv. Ment. Dis.* **164**, 42–50.
60 Harrower, M. R. (1950): The results of psychosomatic and personality tests in multiple sclerosis. *Proc. Assoc. Res. Nerv. Ment. Dis.* **28**, 461–471.
61 Lincoln, N. B. (1981): Discrepancies between capabilities and performance of activities of daily living in multiple sclerosis. *Int. Rehabil. Med.* **3**, 84–88.
62 Kaplan, R. (1984): Substantive and methodological issues in a rating of cognitive and psychological function in multiple sclerosis. *Acta Neurol. Scand.* **101**, 21–28.
63 Peyser, J. M. (1984): Experience in cognitive assessment in MS relevant to developing a simple rating system. *Acta Neurol. Scand.* **101**, 29–31.
64 Zeldow, P. B. & Pavlou, M. (1984): Physical disability, life stress and psychological adjustments in multiple sclerosis. *J. Nerv. Ment. Dis.* **172**, 80–84.
65 Caine, E. D., Bamford, K. A., Schiffer, R. B., Shoulson, I. & Levy, S. (1986): A controlled neuropsychological comparison of Huntington's disease and multiple sclerosis. *Arch. Neurol.* **43**, 249–254.
66 Riklan, M., Levitan, E. & Diller, L. (1961): Psychologic studies in neurologic disease—a review: Parkinson's disease and multiple sclerosis. *J. Am. Geriatr. Soc.* **9**, 857–867.
67 Canter, A. (1951): MMPI profiles in multiple sclerosis. *J. Consult. Psychol.* **44**, 253–256.
68 Ross, A. T. & Reitan, R. M. (1955): Intellectual and affective functions in multiple sclerosis. *A.M.A. Arch. Neurol. Psychiatry* **73**, 663–677.

69 Cleeland, C. S., Matthews, C. G. & Hopper, C. L. (1970): MMPI profiles in exacerbations and remission of multiple sclerosis. *Psychol. Rep.* **27**, 373–374.
70 Peyser, J. M., Edwards, M. R. & Poser, C. M. (1980): Psychological profiles in patients with multiple sclerosis. *Arch. Neurol.* **37**, 437–440.
71 Marsh, G. G., Hirsch, S. H. & Leung, G. (1982): Use and misuse of the MMPI in multiple sclerosis. *Psychol. Rep.* **51**, 1127–1134.
72 Wilson, H, Olson, W., Gascon, G. G. & Brumbach, R. A. (1982): Personality characteristics and multiple sclerosis. *Psychol. Rep.* **51**, 791–806.
73 Davis, L. J., Osborne, D., Siemens, P. J. & Brown, J. R. (1971): MMPI correlates with disability in multiple sclerosis. *Psychol. Rep.* **28**, 700–702.
74 Bergin, J. D. (1957): Rapidly progressing dementia in disseminated sclerosis. *J. Neurol. Neurosurg. Psychiatry.* **20**, 285–292.
75 Braceland, F. J. & Giffin, M. E. (1950): The mental changes associated with multiple sclerosis. *Proc. Assoc. for Research in Nerv. Ment. Dis.* **28**, 450–455.
76 Cremiux, M. M. A, Alliez, J., Togar, M. & Pache, R. (1959); Sclérose en plaque à début par troubles Mentoux. *Rev. Neurol.* **101**, 45–51.
77 Gallinech, A. & Kalinovski, L. B. (1958): Psychiatric aspects of multiple sclerosis. *Diseases of the nervous system* **19**, 77–80.
78 Geocaris, K. (1957): Psychotic episodes heralding the diagnosis of multiple sclerosis. *Bull. Menninger Clin.* **21**, 107–116.
79 Parker, N. (1956): Disseminated sclerosis presenting as schizophrenia. *Med. J. Aust.* **1**, 405–407.
80 Schmaltzbach, O. (1954): Disseminated sclerosis in schizophrenia. *Med. J. Aust.* **1**, 451–452.
81 Pommé, B., Girard, J. & Planche, R. (1963): Forme dépression de début d'une sclérose en plaque. *Ann. Med. Psychol.* **1**, 133.
82 Bignami, A., Gherardi, D. & Gallo, G. (1961): Sclerosi a placche acuta a locallizzatione ipotalamica con sintomatologia psichica di tipo malicomico. *Revista di Neurologia* **31**, 240–268.
83 Koenig, H. (1968): Dementia associated with the benign form of multiple sclerosis. *Trans. Am. Neurol. Assoc.* **93**, 227–228.
84 Mûr, J., Kümpel, G. & Postal, S. (1966): An anergic phase of disseminated sclerosis with psychiatric course. *Confin. Neurol.* **28**, 37–49.
85 Matthews, W. B. (1979): Multiple sclerosis presenting with acute remitting psychiatric symptoms. *J. Neurol. Neurosurg. Psychiatry.* **42**, 859–863.
86 Hollender, M. H. & Stechler, P. P. (1972): Multiple sclerosis and schizophrenia: a case report. *Psychiatry in Medicine* **3**, 251–257.
87 Goodstein, R. K. & Ferrell, R. B. (1977): Multiple sclerosis: presenting as depressive illness. *Diseases of the Nervous System* **38**, 127–131.
88 Caplan, L. R. & Nadelson, T. (1980): Multiple sclerosis and hysteria. *J.A.M.A.* **243**, 2418–2420.
89 Drake, M. E. (1984): Acute paranoid psychosis in multiple sclerosis. *Psychosomatics* **29**, 60–61, 65.
90 Giordana, R., Volpe, G., Tombato, E. & Tavolato, B. (1982): Sindroma dimenziale sintomatica di sclerosi multipla. *Rivista di Neurologia* **52**, 24–32.
91 Kellner, C. H., Davenport, Y., Post, R. M. & Ross, R. J. (1984): Rapidly cycling bipolar disorder and multiple sclerosis. *Am. J. Psychiatry* **41**, 112–113.
92 Surridge, D. (1969): An investigation into some psychiatric aspects of multiple sclerosis. *Br. J. Psychiatry* **115**, 749–764.
93 von Barylla, F. (1961): Zur Invalidisierung Multiple-Sklerose-Kranken unter Berücksichtigungen Psychischer Veränderungen. *Psychiatrie, Neurologie und Medizinische Psychologie* **13**, 443–450.
94 Sai-Halasz, A. (1956): Psychic alterations in disseminated sclerosis. A general, statistical and Rohrschach-test study on 200 patients. *Monatsschrift für Psychiatrie und Neurologia* **132**, 129–154.
95 Mei-Tal, V., Meyerowitz, S. & Engel, G. L. (1970): The role of psychological process in a somatic disorder: Multiple sclerosis. *Psychosom. Med.* **32**, 67–86.
96 Philippopoulos, G. S., Whitthower, E. D. & Cousineau, A. (1958): The etiologic significance of emotional factors in onset and exacerbations of multiple sclerosis. *Psychosom. Med.* **20**, 458–474.

97 Baretz, R. M. & Stephenson, G. R. (1981): Emotional response to multiple sclerosis. *Psychosomatics* **22**, 117–127.
98 Warren, S. W., Greenhill, S. & Warren, K. G. (1982): Emotional stress and the development of multiple sclerosis: case-control evidence of a relationship. *J. Chron. Dis.* **35**, 821–831.
99 McIvor, G. P., Riklan, M. & Reznikoff, M. (1984): Depression in multiple sclerosis as a function of length and severity of illness, age, remissions, and perceived social support. *J. Clin. Psychol.* **40**, 1028–1033.
100 Whitlock, F. A. & Siskind, M. M. (1980): Depression as a major symptom of multiple sclerosis. *J. Neurol. Neurosurg. Psychiatry* **43**, 861–865.
101 Schiffer, R. B., Caine, E. D., Bamford, K. A. & Levy, S. (1983): Depressive episodes in patients with multiple sclerosis. *Am. J. Psychiatry* **140**, 1498–1500.
102 Schiffer, R. B., Winemann, N. M. & Weitkamp, L. R. (1986): Association between bipolar and affective disorder and multiple sclerosis. *Am. J. Psychiatry* **143**, 94–95.
103 Schiffer, R. B. (1987): The spectrum of depression in multiple sclerosis. *Arch. Neurol.* **44**, 596–599.
104 Schiffer, R. B. & Barbigian, M. B. (1984): Behavioral disorders in multiple sclerosis, temporal lobe epilepsy and amyotrophic lateral sclerosis. *Arch. Neurol.* **41**, 1067–1069.
105 Korkina, M. V. *et al.* (1983): Mental disorders in multiple sclerosis. *Zh. Neuropathol. Psikhiatr.* **83**, 732–737.
106 Hower, W. G., Hurwitz, T., Li, D. K. B., Palmer, M. & Paty, D. W. (1987): Temporal lobe involvement in multiple sclerosis patients with psychiatric disorders. *Arch. Neurol.* **44**, 187–190.
107 Bernard, R. O. & Triggs, M. (1974): Corpus callosum in multiple sclerosis. *J. Neurol. Neurosurg. Psychiatry* **37**, 1259–1264.

I

COGNITIVE SCREENING

2

SCREENING MULTIPLE SCLEROSIS PATIENTS FOR COGNITIVE IMPAIRMENT

Michael E. Mahler, R. Jeffrey Davis, and D. Frank Benson

Reed Neurological Research Center; University of California Los Angeles School of Medicine; 710 Westwood Plaza; Los Angeles, California, USA

Summary

A Quick Mental Status Examination (QMSE) has been designed to screen for cognitive impairments in a wide variety of neurological and psychiatric patients. The initial results in multiple sclerosis (MS) patients revealed that 50 percent scored lower than the lowest score registered by normal controls matched for age, sex and education. The QMSE detects clinically significant cognitive impairment in a large subgroup of MS patients and correlates reasonably well with other measures of dysfunction. This method of mental status assessment is easily and rapidly administered, and offers considerable potential as a screening procedure for cognitive impairment in MS patients.

Introduction

Although Charcot[1] described mental enfeeblement in his seminal writings on multiple sclerosis (MS), until recently most clinical references[2] suggested that cognitive impairment was rare and almost only occurred with advanced disease. However, systematic studies using neuropsychometric techniques have demonstrated that neuropsychological deficits are prevalent in MS, and suggest that 25 to 50 percent of patients have some degree of intellectual difficulty.[3] The discrepancy between the low rate of recognition of cognitive disturbances by clinical observers and the high rate of detection by neuropsychological testing has at least two possible explanations. First, many clinicians conceptualize cognitive impairment as being equivalent to dementia of the type seen in Alzheimer's disease; they are not prepared to appreciate the less severe and different pattern of impairment that can be detected in MS patients. Second, the routine mental status examination performed clinically is not adequate for detecting the deficits that occur most often in MS.

Neuropsychometric testing is sensitive and useful for the quantification and full delineation of selected cognitive impairments. The test batteries are time-consuming, require specially trained personnel, are expensive, and are impractical for the initial detection and serial evaluations of those patients with cognitive deficits. A need exists for a screening examination that can be used in a clinical setting, in the office or at the bedside, to identify those patients with the greatest likelihood of having significant cognitive impairment. The requirements of a screening examination are: (1) it must be relatively brief and simple to administer; (2) it must be valid and reliable; and (3) it must be sensitive enough to detect nearly all those in the susceptible population who have intellectual difficulties. In this report, we describe our initial results in MS patients using the Quick Mental Status Examination (QMSE), a screening test of mental status.

Methods

Twenty MS patients were recruited from an outpatient clinic. All were residing at home in their communities, with disability ranging from mild to moderately severe. A control group of volunteers was recruited, consisting of twenty normal residents of the community matched with the MS patients by sex, age, and educational level (See Table 1).

Each MS patient was given two different versions of the QMSE (described below) on separate occasions within one week. In the first session, the full QMSE was administered and in the second session, a social worker administered an abbreviated version of the QMSE. The control subjects were given only the full test. Subjects were aware of the nature of the research and consented to participate.

The QMSE is a brief but broad mental status examination based upon the clinical neurobehaviour examination utilized at U.C.L.A., with a selection of those items that are most discriminating. The test is quantitative, with easy scoring of each item on the test worksheet.

The QMSE contains questions concerning orientation to time and place; forward and reverse span using letters of the alphabet; ten word list memory task using four repetitions of the list and a five minute delay prior to free recall; 'cognition' questions (simple and complex arithmetical calculations, abstraction of verbal similarities and differences, idiomatic expressions, and proverbs); an assessment of language (comprehension, naming, category word generation, repetition, reading, writing); and visuospatial assessment (figure copying). The complete QMSE can be administered in 20 minutes or less and the abbreviated version takes less than 10 minutes. The abbreviated QMSE used for this study contained letter sequences for span determination, a 10 word list for memory determination, and a set of cognition questions. The letter sequences, word lists, and cognitive questions were different but equivalent to the QMSE test items.

In a separate study, the QMSE was given simultaneously with the Mini-Mental State Examination (MMSE)[4] to a different group of 23 patients from the MS clinic to compare performance on these two brief mental status assessment instruments.

Differences between group means were analysed using the Student's *t* test. Correlations were analysed through the use of a regression coefficient.

Results

The results are shown in Tables 1 and 2. The patient and control groups each consisted of 16 women and four men. Although the controls were slightly younger (mean age 43.6 years *vs* 46.7) and better educated (13.6 years *vs* 13.2) these differences were not significant.

Table 1. *QMSE results in multiple sclerosis patients and normal controls.* Results are means (s.d.).

Variable	*MS patients (n = 20)*[a]	*Controls (n = 20)*[a]
Age (years)	46.7 (12.4)	43.6 (12.9)*
range	35–69	32–70
Education (duration in years)	13.2 (2.8)	13.6 (2.1)*
Total QMSE (maximum 100, with 2 free points)	75.0 (10.5)	89.0 (4.2)†
Orientation (maximum 5)	5.0 (0.2)	5.0 (0.1)*
Forward span (maximum 6)	4.9 (0.9)	6.0 (1.1)†
Reverse span (maximum 6)	2.6 (0.8)	4.4 (0.7)†
Memory (maximum 30)	20.0 (4.9)	23.4 (2.7)§
Cognition (maximum 15)	10.0 (4.1)	13.6 (3.4)†
Language (maximum 24)	22.8 (1.5)	23.4 (1.4)*
Constructions (maximum 12)	10.1 (1.8)	11.0 (1.3)*

[a]female:male 16:4
*difference not significant
†$P < 0.005$ *vs* control
§$P < 0.01$ *vs* control

The maximum score on the QMSE is 100 points. Based on our experience using the QMSE in a variety of neurological conditions, we have determined that a score below 80 is indicative of significant cognitive difficulty. The mean total score of the MS group was 75 (s.d. 10.5), while the mean score of the control group was 89 (4.2), a striking and statistically significant ($P < 0.005$) difference. The lowest control subject score was 81; only six MS patients scored higher than 80.

The MS patients performed poorly on the forward and reverse letter sequences, the difference in comparison to the control group being significant at the 0.005 level. The difference between scores on both the immediate and delayed recall portion of the memory task was also significant ($P < 0.01$ for the combined memory score). There were no differences between the groups on the scores for the orientation section or for the language section, both patients and controls scoring nearly perfectly.

The coefficient of correlation between the full QMSE scores and the scores obtained with the abbreviated test administered to the MS patients a few days later was $r = 0.72$. When the scores of the forward and reverse sequences and the word learning task were combined, this subtotal correlated well with the total QMSE score, $r = 0.9$.

Twenty-three MS patients were tested with both the QMSE and the MMSE. They had a mean score of 28 out of a possible 30 points. On the MMSE, a score of 24 or less is considered impaired. Only one patient scored below this level. The mean QMSE for this group was 74, and 10 patients scored below 80. Seven of the 10 low-scoring patients had Kurtzke scores of 8 or 9, indicating severe disability. Of 13 patients with Kurtzke scores between 2 and 7, 10 scored over 80.

Table 2. *QMSE compared to MMSE in 23 multiple sclerosis patients.*

	MMSE > 24	*MMSE < 25*	*Totals*
QMSE > 80	13	0	13
QMSE < 81	9	1	10
Totals	22	1	23

Discussion

The mean scores of the MS patients were significantly different from those of the matched control group for the QMSE as a whole and for many of the subtests. The most prominent differences were found on the forward and reverse span sequences and the memory task. Half the MS patients scored lower than the lowest control, in a range indicative of clinically significant impairment.

The abbreviated version of the QMSE correlated highly with the full version and this can be taken as a measure of test-retest reliability. It also suggests that this abbreviated assessment instrument represents a useful tool for screening MS patients for cognitive impairment. The QMSE, either in its full or abbreviated form, appears to be superior to another commonly used brief mental status test, the MMSE.

The QMSE scores showed a rough correlation with the Kurtzke disability score, with more disabled patients showing greater cognitive impairment.

The percentage of patients scoring in the impaired range is roughly equal to the proportion detected by others with an extended series of neuropsychometric tests. The pattern of impairment seen with the two assessment techniques, ie neuropsychological batteries and the QMSE, is also similar, with deficits occurring in the areas of memory and concentration in both, but with sparing of language function. This pattern is similar to that seen with subcortical dementing processes.[5] In MS, the primary site of cerebral pathology is in the deep white matter, especially in the periventricular regions; it is not surprising that the subcortical pattern of cognitive impairment seen in the AIDS-dementia complex,[6] Binswanger's disease, and other white matter disease,[7] is also seen in MS.

Based on this brief evaluation the QMSE appears to hold considerable promise as a screening test for mental impairment in MS but it will be necessary to extend the normative data base, to assess further the test-retest reliability, and to validate the test with more extensive clinical and neuropsychometric data.

Acknowledgements—The authors appreciate the efforts of Diana Kramer, MD, and Christine Donovan, M.S.W., in collecting portions of the data, and the referrals of patients by George Ellison, M.D., and Lawrence Meyers, M.D. This work was supported by the Veterans Administration and by a National Institute on Aging Academic Award to Dr. Mahler. The United States and Denmark Multiple Sclerosis Societies also provided support.

References

1 Charcot, J. M. (1877): *Lectures on the diseases of the nervous system delivered at La Salpetriere*, pp 195–195. London: New Sydenham Society.

2 McKhan, G. M. (1982): Multiple sclerosis. *Ann. Rev. Neurosci.* **5**, 219–239.

3 Rao, S. M. (1986): Neuropsychology of multiple sclerosis: a critical review. *J. Clin. Exp. Neuropsychol.* **8**, 503–542.

4 Folstein, M. F., Folstein, S. E. & McHugh, P. R. (1975): "Mini-mental state": a practical method for grading the cognitive state of patients for the clinician. *J. Psychiatr. Res.* **12**, 189–198.

5 Cummings, J. L. (1986): Subcortical dementia: neuropsychology, neuropsychiatry, and pathophysiology. *Br. J. Psychiatry* **149**, 682–697.

6 Navia, B. A., Jordan, B. D. & Price, R. W. (1986): The AIDS dementia complex. I. Clinical features. *Ann. Neurol.* **19**, 517–524.

7 Mahler, M. E., Cummings, J. L. & Tomiyasu, U. (1987): Atypical dementia syndrome in an elderly male. *J. Am. Geriatr. Soc.* **35**, 1116–1126.

II

COGNITIVE DEFICITS

3

NEUROPSYCHOLOGICAL IMPAIRMENT IN EARLY MULTIPLE SCLEROSIS

I. Grant, W. Ian McDonald* and M. R. Trimble*

*San Diego VA Medical Center and Department of Psychiatry University of California (San Diego) School of Medicine and *Institute of Neurology, National Hospital, Queen Square, London, UK*

Summary

Neuropsychological impairment has been well documented among patients with advanced multiple sclerosis, but information on cognitive disturbance in the early phases of this disease continues to be fragmentary. In this chapter we review evidence for deficiencies in learning and memory in the early and middle phases of multiple sclerosis. Both short-term and long-term memory impairments have been noted, and these appear to involve both verbal and visual skills. Tests of psychomotor speed and flexibility of thinking (eg, Trail Making Tests) may also show early impairment. Data from a seven-year clinical outcome study suggest that performance on the Trail Making Tests is predictive of future disability as measured by Kurtzke disability status.

Introduction and background

In the latter half of the nineteenth century those clinicians whose pioneering work defined multiple sclerosis much as we understand it today already appreciated that intellectual impairment, and memory loss in particular, were frequent accompaniments of the disorder. Charcot's lectures noted that 'there is marked enfeeblement of memory; conceptions are formed slowly; the intellectual and emotional faculties are blunted in their totality.'[1] German authors of the period also observed that there could be difficulties with memory and in other intellectual domains.[2]

Despite this early recognition that higher mental functions could be impaired in multiple sclerosis, progress in defining the prevalence, qualitative features, and natural history of cognitive decline have been slow in coming. For example, the 1922 report by Brown & Davis simply stated that mental deterioration was present in the majority of cases.[3] Indeed, for a time there was some controversy as to whether cognitive impairment was an important feature of multiple sclerosis. In 1926 Cottrell & Wilson[4] reported that only two of their hundred patients with multiple sclerosis had intellectual deterioration. Instead, these authors focused on the importance of eutonia, a sense of inappropriate physical well being, present in 84 percent of their cases, and euphoria, which they found in 63 percent. A later study by Sugar & Nadell[5] also failed to note any substantial rate of intellectual impairment.

The first author to attempt a prevalence estimate appears to have been Ombredane[6] whose thesis to the University of Paris reported that 72 percent of his 50 patients with MS suffered from some intellectual deficiency. Six of these (12%) were so severely impaired as to be classified demented; the remaining 30 (60%) had intellectual deficits which included 'difficulté de l'effort intellectuel' and 'l'affaiblissment de la memoire'. In terms of memory difficulties, the least affected was 'memoire des faits anciens appertenant à la vie personnelle du malade' and the most affected was 'memoire de fixation', which we may take to mean recent learning. Ombredane also noted visual-spatial difficulties—eg map reading. He noted deficits also in 'les fonctions d'analyse et de synthese'.

A more precise delineation of the frequency and features of cognitive change in multiple sclerosis had to await the development of neuropsychological techniques, beginning in the 1940s, and it was not until 1955 that the first reasonably comprehensive neuropsychological study of multiple sclerosis was reported by Ross & Reitan.[16] These authors found substantial impairments in complex perceptual motor skills in the majority of patients, some deficiency in abstract meaning, and generally preserved verbal intellectual skills. Most of the work which has followed has generally confirmed this overall pattern of deficits.[2,7]

Present neuropsychological research is attempting to characterize the process of breakdown in cognitive function as well as to relate neuropsychological impairments to neuropathological findings as visualized on magnetic resonance imaging (MRI) and to overall progress in clinical disability. In this chapter we shall review some of our own data on neuropsychological deficiency in early multiple sclerosis, and present some preliminary observations on attempts to predict future clinical decline from initial neuropsychological test results.

The first large series of MS patients to undergo a formal memory assessment was reported by Jambor.[8] The typical patient was examined 6–10 years after diagnosis. Assessments included Babcock sentences and a task involving delayed recall of pictures. Compared to muscular dystrophy controls, patients with MS required more trials to learn sentences and also had impaired picture recall.

Beatty & Gange[9] used list learning as their paradigm. A series of 26 patients whose average length of disease was 9 years was assessed. Patients were presented with a list of 24 words over four trials. The authors found that patients' learning over the four trials was less efficient than that of controls. Furthermore, patients also scored worse on a delayed recall task based on multiple choice questions about a short story presented 30 minutes before.

Staples & Lincoln[10] used the Wechsler Memory Scale (WMS—original version) to assess attention and memory in a more comprehensive fashion. The performance of 29 MS patients with moderately advanced disease (average duration of illness = 15.9 years) was compared to that of patients with muscular dystrophy. The authors found that MS patients were inferior on delayed recall of both WMS stories and figures compared to the neuromuscular group. On initial learning, however, MS patients were worse only on figure learning; they were indistinguishable from the muscular dystrophy patients on immediate story memory.

The possibility that MS patients might have more difficulty in visual than verbal memory has not received systematic support. For example, Carroll *et al.*[11] came to the opposite conclusion—that MS patients had more difficulty with a verbal recognition test than with picture recognition. These same authors postulated that MS patients might have particular difficulties in what they termed 'relational' processing, ie, being able to form semantic categories which facilitate the recall of information which can be grouped logically. In their study patients were expected to recognize previously presented 'familiar' and 'unfamiliar' words. Patients with MS had more difficulty than controls with 'familiar' word recognition, while being roughly equivalent on the 'unfamiliar' task. Controls appeared to form logical semantic groupings more easily which facilitated their recall of 'familiar' words, whereas patients with MS had more difficulties with forming such groupings and, indeed, their efforts sometimes resulted in inter-item semantic encoding confusion.

Some of the most extensive work on learning and memory in MS has been conducted by Rao and associates.[12] In their initial studies these investigators administered the Wechsler Memory Scale (original version) and a word list learning task to 44 patients with chronic MS. Comparison subjects included a group of 23 pain patients and 15 hospital workers. The word list learning paradigm consisted of presentation of a series of words over five trials, followed by a distractor list, then a short-term free recall of the original list, and finally a 30 minute delayed recall. A spatial recall task using a similar paradigm was also employed. The authors found that MS patients were impaired on verbal and non-verbal learning and recall compared to non-patient controls, but that there were fewer differences on the verbal recall procedure when MS patients were compared to pain patients. Thus retrieval of non-verbal information appeared to suffer particularly, echoing back to the earlier observations of Staples & Lincoln.[10]

The results of several new studies were presented in a preliminary fashion at the conference in Odense which focused specifically on neuropsychiatric correlates of multiple sclerosis. At this meeting Lyon-Caen *et al.* (this volume, chapter 15) noted that 46 percent of 50 patients with acute optic neuritis or early multiple sclerosis (less than 2 years duration) had neuropsychological impairment in a battery of tests which included Wisconsin Card Sorting, WAIS, story and figure learning and recall, and fluency. In terms of memory, both verbal and non-verbal impairments were seen, whereas verbal fluency (which can be equated to long-term semantic memory) was normal. Fischer (this volume, chapter 5) reported on data from the Cleveland clinic where 45 patients with definite multiple sclerosis received the revised version of the Wechsler Memory Scale (WMS-R). MS patients were impaired relative to education-matched non-patient controls on all five indices of the WMS-R, their most striking impairments being on the delayed recall index. A cluster analytic approach led to the identification of three possible clusters including a group of 11 patients with normal memory, 25 with mild impairments in learning and recall, and the remainder with generalized moderate to severe impairments in short-term memory learning and long-term memory. Stenager and colleagues (this volume, chapter 4) reported on 115 patients with definite MS with a broad range of disabilities as assessed by the Kurtzke Functional Scale. These investigators observed that even among patients who were functionally quite intact (Kurtzke scale scores of 1 and 2) performance on story recall was significantly worse when compared to healthy controls. Rao (this volume, chapter 8) presented the results of his group's on-going studies which confirmed defects in retrieval of both verbal and non-verbal information among patients with multiple sclerosis. Interestingly, Rao did not find short-term memory problems, based on a Peterson word trigram procedure, which contrasts with some of our findings as will be seen below.

In summary, observations to date suggest that at least half of an unselected group of patients with multiple sclerosis will show some impairment in neuropsychological functioning. Defects in verbal and non-verbal learning and recall are commonly found, though relationship to progression of illness has been established less firmly. One of the purposes of the study which we performed, and describe below, was to determine whether disturbances in learning and recall could be identified relatively early in the natural history of multiple sclerosis. In the description which follows, we shall review some of the findings from our original study[13] and present some new analyses based on a follow-up of the records of 34 of the original 43 subjects.

Investigation of neuropsychological impairment

Subjects

*Original MS cohort (*n = *43).* Of these 43 patients 29 were inpatients and 14 were outpatients at the National Hospitals, Queen Square or Maida Vale. There were 31 patients with clinically definite MS, 11 with probable MS, and one with early progressive disease in the original sample. Twenty six patients were tested within 5 years of diagnosis, 13 at 6 to 10 years, and four at 11 to 15 years post-diagnosis. Thus, the majority represented relatively early MS, and the number of 'years of active disease' (number of years in which the patient reported at least one week's duration of symptoms) was 4.5 ± 3.6.

Non-patient controls. We selected 17 women and 11 men roughly to parallel the sex distribution of the MS patients and matched them as closely as possible on age and estimated intelligence based on the WAIS vocabulary scale score (Table 1).

*MS patients whose records were followed up 7 years later (*n = *34).* Approximately 6 to 7 years after initial examination it was possible to perform a records review of patients who were studied originally. At this writing thirty-four of the original 43 records (79%) could be located and contained sufficient follow-up information upon which to base a judgment of functional status (Kurtzke functional rating scale) at one year or more after initial examination. In terms of age, education, vocabulary scale score and years of active disease, these patients were comparable to the original sample using information gathered at baseline (t-test, all $P > 0.05$).

Procedures

Neuropsychological testing. At initial evaluation all patients received the WAIS-R vocabulary test, Trail Making Tests parts A and B, Wechsler Memory Scale (original) story ('American Liner, New York') and figures using Heaton's modification. Briefly, the latter two involve reading the story or presenting the figures with an immediate recall required after 10 seconds. If at least 15 elements of the story (or figures) are not recalled using Heaton's scoring system, then the story or figures are presented again up to five times in an effort to reach the criterion. A 45 minute delayed recall was also used, allowing for the following scores to be computed: initial recall; number of trials needed to reach criterion; and delayed recall.

We also administered the Brown Peterson test using consonant trigrams according to the method described by Butters *et al.*[17] This involved presentation of 30 trigrams randomized across three rehearsal conditions (0, 2 and 4 seconds delay) and five interference conditions (0, 3, 6, 9 and 18 seconds of counting backwards by threes).

Table 1. *Age and Vocabulary Scale Score of subjects.*

	MS patients (initial evaluation)	*MS patients (7 year follow-up of records)*	*Non-patient controls*
Number	43	34	28
Age (s.d.)	37.8 (10.2)	37.7 (10.1)	34.8 (10.3)
Vocabulary Scale score (s.d.)	11.9 (2.3)	12.1 (2.1)	12.3 (2.7)

Disability status rating. As noted above, in 34 of the original 43 cases medical records were available which included follow-up information of sufficient quality at least one year after the initial evaluation to enable us to make a disability rating using the Kurtzke Expanded Disability Status Scale.[18] The median length of follow-up was 6 years with a range of 1 to 7 years. Since disability ratings were available both for the initial evaluation and for the last follow-up medical visit, it was possible to compute a Kurtzke status difference score to reflect change in status in the interim. For some analyses described below, patients who deteriorated by one full step or more were classified as substantially worsened ($n = 15$) whilst, the rest ($n = 19$) were termed unchanged (which included the few cases who showed some improvement).

Results

Neuropsychological performance at initial assessment

Table 2 shows average neuropsychological test results for patients compared with non-patients at initial evaluation. Very substantial differences are evident on Trail Making part A and B, here probably reflecting the MS patients' psychomotor slowing. At the same time patients exhibit significant difficulties in initial learning of both verbal and non-verbal information (trial 1 of story or figures), require more trials to master visual and verbal material (trials to criterion score), and tend to forget more of the initially learned material after a 45 minute delay.

Interestingly, these difficulties with learning and remembering are also expressed on a test traditionally thought to measure short-term memory, or what Rao has termed 'primary

Table 2. *Learning and memory in multiple sclerosis: neuropsychological test results.* Data are means (s.d.)

	Groups		*Statistics*	
Tests	*Patients* n = *43*	*Non-patients* n = *28*	*F(1,69)*	*P<*
Trail Making				
Part A (time-second)	51.4 (25.8)	27.9 (9.3)	21.0	0.0001
Part B (time-second)	105.8 (56.3)	65.7 (22.8)	12.6	0.001
WMS story				
Trial 1 (no. of bits)	8.4 (3.4)	12.6 (3.8)	23.0	0.0001
Trials to criterion	3.2 (1.3)	1.9 (0.6)	26.3	0.0001
45 minute delay	13.5 (2.9)	16.6 (3.0)	19.7	0.0001
WMS Figures				
Trial 1 (no. of bits)	13.6 (4.3)	17.0 (2.8)	13.7	0.001
Trials to criterion	2.1 (1.3)	1.0 (0.2)	16.9	0.0001
45 minute delay	15.0 (3.9)	16.8 (2.8)	4.21	0.05
Brown-Peterson				
Total % correct	59.3 (19.0)	69.8 (21.1)	4.77	0.04
No interference	98.6 (6.4)	95.2 (8.9)	4.19	0.05*
Interference	49.6 (23.0)	63.9 (25.4)	6.06	0.02
No delay	45.3 (25.9)	57.6 (29.7)	3.37	NS
4 second delay	52.9 (26.3)	62.1 (28.8)	1.91	NS

*Multiple sclerosis patients better

memory'. The disturbance seemed to occur primarily when patients were required to learn in the face of distraction. While the opportunity to rehearse free of interference for up to 4 seconds seemed to improve performance somewhat, this benefit was not sufficient to offset the subsequent disruption of encoding produced by pro-active interference.

Table 3 summarizes the results of a series of multiple regression studies which attempted to predict performance on each neuropsychological test from a set of independent variables that included years of active disease, age, education, and active/quiescent status (ie, whether the person was going through an exacerbation or not at the time of testing). These stepwise regressions indicate that length of active disease accounts for most of the variability in psychomotor performance (here measured by Trails A and B), whilst performance on the Brown Peterson procedure seems to reflect the joint influences not only of years of active disease but also whether the patient was experiencing an exacerbation at time of testing, as well as the expected influence of age and education. A separate set of regression studies (not presented in the Table) in which current medication with ACTH or steroids was substituted as a variable for education failed to reveal any significant effect of medication status on neuropsychological test scores.

Disability outcome in relation to initial neuropsychological status

The median follow-up for the records review was 6 years (1 to 7 years). The median score for these 34 patients was 3.0 (range 1 to 8.5) on the Kurtzke Expanded Disability Status Scale at initial examination. At follow-up the median disability status was 3.5 (range 0 to 10) and the median change from baseline was 0.5 steps (range −3.0 to 4.5, a negative score signifying improvement in status).

From the above it can be seen that whereas the group's central tendency was to undergo a slight deterioration during the 6 year follow-up, there was considerable variability with

Table 3. *Learning and memory in multiple sclerosis.* Predicting test performance with years of active disease age, acute/quiescent status and education.

	Cumulative % accountable variance[a]				
Dependent measures	*Years of active disease*	*Age*	*Education*	*Active quiescent status*	*F(4,38)*
Trailmaking					
Part A	0.50	0.51	0.51	0.51	8.76‡
Part B	0.46	0.46	0.47	0.48	7.66‡
Brown-Peterson					
Total % correct	0.10	0.23	0.33	0.41	6.50†
No interference	0.28	0.28	0.29	0.29	3.80*
9 seconds interference	0.15	0.20	0.30	0.41	6.65†
18 seconds interference	0.01	0.12	0.21	0.22	2.63
WAIS vocabulary	0.08	0.09	0.27	0.34	4.06†

[a]These are cumulative R^2 values and can be read as % variance in test accounted for by addition of each predictor. The R^2 under column 4 is identical to R^2 for the entire multiple regression, where R = multiple correlation. Example for Trails B: years of active disease accounts for 46% of variance in that test; age yields no added predictive power; education adds 1% prediction, and active/quiescent status adds a final 1% for a total $R^2 = 0.48$. The unadjusted multiple R is $\sqrt{0.48}$, or 0.69 for this regression.
*$P<0.05$, †$P<0.01$, ‡$P<0.001$.

a few patients improving and others getting significantly worse. Indeed, two died during the follow-up.

To assess whether any information from initial neuropsychological testing could help predict longer term disability status, we partitioned the sample of 34 cases into those who worsened (ie, who came to occupy at least one step higher on the Kurtzke Disability Status Scale at follow-up) *vs* those who were essentially unchanged or improved.

Table 4 shows the age, education, years of active disease, initial disability status score, and initial neuropsychological test results for the two groups. Patients who underwent a significant deterioration tended to be slightly older, to have an average of almost two more years of active disease, and to be somewhat more disabled at initial evaluation, but none of these differences was statistically significant.

The only significant neuropsychological difference was on Trail Making part B. Patients who later deteriorated had significantly more cognitive/psychomotor impairment based on this measure at initial testing than those who remained unchanged or improved.

In an effort to determine whether a group of characteristics, in concert, might significantly predict follow-up disability status we performed a stepwise multiple regression analysis with change in disability as the dependent variable and age, years of active disease, initial Trail Making B score and initial Peterson Consonant Trigram Error score as the predictor variables. (Because of small sample size we deliberately kept the number of variables small, limiting them to some of the more plausible candidates—age and years of disease for obvious reasons, and Trails B and Peterson representing our two major cognitive domains—speed of information processing and memory.) Setting F to enter variables into the equation at 4.0 and F to remove a variable at 3.996, the computation completed only one step, entering one variable—Trails B—before reaching the statistical limit. The multiple R was 0.62 ($R^2=0.38$; adjusted $R^2=0.37$. A second stepwise regression in which initial Kurtzke disability status was substituted for age in the predictor set yielded a higher R but eliminated Trailmaking part B as a significant predictor.

Table 4. *Age, education, years of active disease, disability status, and neuropsychological test score at* initial evaluation *of patients who later either remained unchanged on Kurtzke disability status, or deteriorated.* Results are means (s.d.).

Initial (baseline) characteristic	*Same or better* (n = *19)*	*Worse* (n = *15)*
Age	35.6 (9.4)	40.3 (10.6)
Education	11.7 (2.5)	11.2 (2.4)
Years of active disease	3.3 (1.9)	5.1 (4.2)
Baseline Kurtzke step	2.9 (2.1)	4.3 (2.4)
Vocabulary scale score	12.1 (2.4)	12.1 (1.8)
Peterson total correct (out of 30 max)	19.6 (5.5)	16.3 (6.1)
Story learning, trials to criterion	2.8 (1.5)	3.4 (1.5)
Trail Making B	84.1 (42.8)*	129.3 (69.0)*

*$t=2.35$, $P<0.03$

Frequency of impairment in memory and other cognitive functions at various disability levels

We also examined the relationship of initial neuropsychological test results to initial disability level to try to get an idea of the prevalence of two forms of neuropsychological impairment, ie, impairment in memory and impairment in speed of information processing, as measured by the Trail Making Test, at different Kurtzke steps. The 34 cases were classified as minimally disabled (Kurtzke steps 0, 1, 2), mildly to moderately disabled (Kurtzke steps 3, 4, 5), moderately to severely disabled (Kurtzke steps 6, 7), and very severely disabled (Kurtzke steps 8, 9). A six point impairment rating scale was created for the group of memory tests and a similar scale for the pair of Trail Making Tests. In this scale a rating of 1 indicated exceptionally good performance, 2 = average, 3 = atypical, 4 = definite mild impairment, 5 = moderate impairment, and 6 = severe impairment.

The figure shows the relationship of median impairment scores for memory and the psychomotor variable (Trail Making Tests) to disability group assignment. It can be seen that there is an almost linear progression from normal to severely impaired across the Kurtzke groupings. Interestingly, even the minimally impaired patients at Kurtzke steps 0, 1, and 2 already achieve a median impairment rating of 3 (atypical) for memory. These data tend to reinforce our previous observation that subtle memory changes can occur rather early in the course of multiple sclerosis, earlier even than the sorts of psychomotor inefficiencies that might be reflected in deteriorated Trail making performance.

Conclusions

In the past two decades there has been a substantial increment in our understanding of the neuropsychological correlates of multiple sclerosis. It has become clear that deficiency in learning and memory can occur early in the course of the disease, even whilst patients are only very mildly symptomatic from a neurological standpoint and when their disability level is low.

There continues to be some divergence of opinion as to the nature of memory loss in multiple sclerosis. According to Rao,[15] the defects are principally in 'secondary memory'

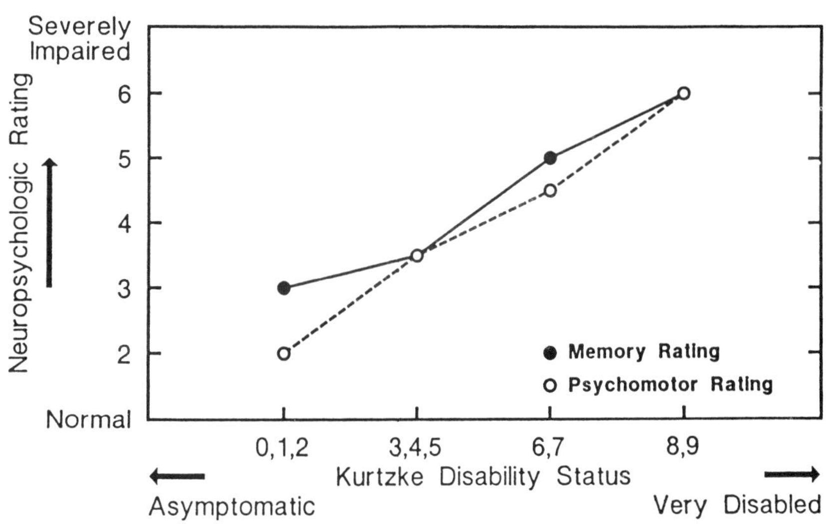

Figure. *Relation of memory rating and psychomotor rating to disability status in MS patients (n = 34).*

which most neuropsychologists would equate to a deficit in retrieval. Our own data suggest that there may be a broader form of memory deficit which spans encoding, short-term recall, and longer term retrieval. It may be that the inconsistencies of our findings and those of Rao on the Peterson paradigm reflect differences in level of difficulty in tasks chosen—we believe that the consonant trigrams are inherently more taxing and may reveal subtle defects in short-term memory which word trigrams (the paradigm used by Rao and associates) failed to detect.

We think it unlikely that patients with MS have specific deficiencies in visual memory as compared to verbal memory, as suggested in the data of Staples & Lincoln.[10] As we noted above, some authors (eg Carroll *et al.*[11]) actually found the opposite to be true, whereas our own data suggest that encoding and retrieval of figural and verbal information are both affected to about the same extent.

Some of the newer data presented here also suggest that there may be differential progression of neuropsychological deficits with course of disease. As demonstrated in the Figure, it appears that subtle memory defects can occur at very early stages of multiple sclerosis, at a time when other functions, such as the speeded information processing, thought to be measured by the Trail Making Tests, are still normal.

Whereas subtle changes in memory might be the earliest signs of cerebral impairment in multiple sclerosis, they might not be the most important prognostically. Indeed, our multiple regression studies, which attempted to predict disability outcome 6 years after assessing baseline neuropsychological status, indicate that it is performance on the Trail Making Tests, not on memory tests, which is most strongly associated with subsequent functional deterioration.

In conclusion, our data and those of other investigators confirm that memory difficulties are ubiquitous in multiple sclerosis, even at its earliest stages. These findings suggest the importance of careful neuropsychological examination which includes sophisticated assessment of memory in the routine evaluation of patients suspected of having demyelinating disease.

Acknowledgements—This research was supported in part by VA award SA 325 to Dr. I. Grant from the Medical Research Service of the Veterans Administration. The authors thank Michelle Page for her assistance in the preparation of this manuscript.

This chapter appears also in Rao, S. M. (Ed) *Multiple Sclerosis: A Neuropsychological Approach* Oxford University Press (in press). New York: In the public domain.

References

1 Charcot, J. M. (1877): *Lectures on the diseases of the nervous system*. London: New Sydenham Society.

2 Trimble, M. R. & Grant, I. (1982): Psychiatric aspects of multiple sclerosis. In *Psychiatric aspects of neurologic disease*, vol. II, ed D. F. Benson & D. Blumer, pp 279–299. New York: Grune & Stratton.

3 Brown, S. & Davis, T. K. (1922): The mental symptoms of multiple sclerosis. *Arch. Neurol. Psychiatry* **7**, 629–634.

4 Cottrell, S. S. & Wilson, T. K. (1922): The affective symptomatology of multiple sclerosis. *J. Neurol. Psychopathol.* **7**, 1–30.

5 Sugar, C. & Nadell, R. (1943): Mental symptoms in multiple sclerosis: A study of 28 cases with a review of the literature. *J. Nerv. Ment. Dis.* **98**, 267–280.

6 Ombredane, M. A. (1929): Sur les troubles mentaux de la sclerose en plaques pour servir à la determination des facteurs organiques dans les maladies mentales. Paris: Faculté de Médicine de Paris, Thèse pour le doctorat en Médicine.

7 Grant, I. (1986): Neuropsychological and psychiatric disturbances in multiple sclerosis. In *Multiple sclerosis*, ed W. I. McDonald & D. H. Silberberg, pp 134–152. London: Butterworths.
8 Jambor, K. L. (1969): Cognitive functioning in multiple sclerosis. *Br. J. Psychiatry* **115**, 765–775.
9 Beatty, P. A. & Gange, J. J. (1977): Neuropsychological aspects of multiple sclerosis. *J. Nerv. Ment. Dis.* **164**, 42–50.
10 Staples, D. & Lincoln, N. B. (1979): Intellectual impairment in multiple sclerosis. *Rheumatol. Rehab.* **18**, 153–160.
11 Carroll, M., Gates, R. & Roldan, F. (1984): Memory impairment in multiple sclerosis. *Neuropsychologia* **22**, 297–302.
12 Rao, S. M., Hammeke, T. A., McQuillen, M. P., Khatari, B. O. & Lloyd, D. (1984): Memory disturbance in chronic progressive multiple sclerosis. *Arch. Neurol.* **41**, 625–631.
13 Grant, I., McDonald, W. I., Trimble, M. R., Smith, E. & Reed, R. (1984): Deficient learning and memory in early and middle phases of multiple sclerosis. *J. Neurol. Neurosurg. Psychiatry* **57**, 250–255.
14 Butters, E. J. & Velano, T. W. (1978): Auditory and visual cognitive styles and adult reading performance. *Percept. Mot. Skills* **47**, 995–998.
15 Kurtzke, J. S. (1983): Rating neurological impairment in multiple sclerosis: an expanded disability status scale (EDSS). *Neurology* **33**, 1444–1452.
16 Ross, A. T., Reitan, R. M. (1955): Intellectual and affective functions in multiple sclerosis: A quantitative study. *AMA Archives of Neurology and Psychiatry* **73**, 663–677.

4

MULTIPLE SCLEROSIS: CORRELATION OF COGNITIVE DYSFUNCTION WITH KURTZKE DISABILITY STATUS SCALE

Egon Stenager, Lone Knudsen and Knud Jensen

Clinical Neuropsychiatric Research Unit, Departments of Neurology, Clinical Psychology, and Psychiatry, Odense University Hospital, Odense, Denmark

Summary

This study compares 115 multiple sclerosis (MS) patients (age 25–55 years) with definite MS, admitted to the neurological department, Odense University Hospital between April 1973 and December 1985, with healthy controls (n = 39) matched for sex, age and socio-economic status, using a neuropsychological test battery. Cognitive function of the patients was independent of age. In one memory test (story recall) MS patients with even the slightest physical impairment performed significantly worse than the controls. Cognitive dysfunction increased with increasing physical impairment, as measured by the auditive Verbal Learning Test, story recall, Recurring Figure Test, Visual Gestalt Test, Trail Making parts A + B, and the Symbol Digit Modalities Test.

Introduction

The subject of this chapter is the correlation of physical impairment, measured on the Kurtzke Disability Status Scale (KDSS),[1] to cognitive functioning in patients with multiple sclerosis (MS). The patients are also compared with a healthy control group. The tests employed are intelligence tests, memory tests and attention and perceptual motor speed tests.

It can be seen from the literature on this subject that there is some disagreement on whether there is a correlation between the degree of the patients' physical disability and their performance in intelligence tests.[2-4] There is also disagreement on whether there is any correlation between physical disability and performance on memory tests.[5-10] With regard to 'tests of attention and perceptual motor speed' there is agreement that the performance of MS patients is significantly poorer than that of control persons,[3,6] that performance becomes poorer with increasing degree of physical disability[3] and that this decline in performance is conditioned by motor dysfunction[9] and not by inability to concentrate.[5]

We shall first describe our material and methods briefly.

Material and methods

The patients in this investigation were selected from patients with a diagnosis of MS, who were admitted to the Neurological Department, Odense University Hospital, in the period April 1, 1973 to December 31, 1985. In all, there were 463 patients. The following criteria had to be met for inclusion in the investigation: (1) the patients satisfied 'research criteria' as drawn up by Poser *et al.*[11]; (2) they lived in the geographic region of Funen; and (3) their primary language was Danish, because of the neuropsychological tests. Exclusion criteria were: (1) presence of other primary CNS disease; (2) presence of other disease with secondary effects on the CNS; and (3) presence of other chronic disease.

After exclusions, there were 366 patients who satisfied these criteria. To ensure validity in the neuropsychological examination it was decided only to use patients within the age range 25–55 years. As it was not possible to discover from published sources whether the tests were age-dependent for MS patients, the patients were divided into 5 year age groups within the overall age range. As far as possible each age group contained 25 patients. The patients were chosen by random selection.

In the course of the investigation a number of patients withdrew or were excluded for the following reasons: (1) alcohol abuse, arbitrarily defined as more than six drinks daily (none of the patients who remained in the investigation had a regular

Table 1. *Details of patients in the study and exclusions.*

	Age groups (years)				
	25–35	*36–40*	*41–45*	*46–50*	*51–55*
Number of patients included	23	25	21	24	22
Number of patients excluded:					
Poser criteria not fulfilled (see ref[11])	12	5	8	9	12
Residing outside catchment area	10	8	5	8	4
Danish not primary language	1	0	0	0	0
Concurrent disease	2	5	6	2	3
Deceased	1	3	2	1	6
Own physician advised non-involvement	5	3	3	1	1
Patient not willing to participate	2	0	3	2	8
Unable to complete neuro-psychological test	1	0	2	0	1
Unable to establish contact with patient	3	1	1	0	2
Patients excluded by random sampling	0	12	0	6	0
Total number	60	62	51	53	59
Proportion of patients examined (%)	38.3	40.3	41.2	45.3	37.2

daily alcohol consumption); (2) failure to understand the neuropsychological tests or, as a minimum requirement, to cope with the language tests; (3) the patient's general practitioner advised against the examination; (4) refusal to participate; (5) failure to respond to our inquiry.

Table 1 shows how the 115 patients remaining in the investigation were distributed according to age group. Those who were excluded or who dropped out are also classified in this table according to age group and reason for elimination. For these latter patients, the only group which is clearly distinguished from the others is the oldest one; in this group the death frequency and the frequency of those declining to take part was notably greater than in the other groups. Judging from the case histories, those unwilling to take part were those who were the most handicapped. Percentages for those examined varied only slightly from age group to age group and amounted to about 40 percent of the original population. Forty-eight percent of those in the original population suspected of having definite multiple sclerosis were entered into the investigation. Table 2 shows that the male/female ratio in the groups was similar, apart from the oldest group, where it was particularly the women who did not wish to participate.

Table 3 shows the characteristics of the patients in the investigation. It can be seen that, apart from the youngest group, the distribution of disabilities was uniform. As could be expected, the youngest had the fewest disabilities. All patients had definite MS, according to the criteria of Poser *et al.* The patients are grouped according to social status following the criteria used by the Institute for Danish Social Research, in which both education and social status in society is taken into account. For the patients with MS, social status prior to onset of the disease, or the highest status achieved, is used. The table also shows that the social status distribution was uniform for all the age groups. Finally it can be seen that the time interval from self-reported first symptom to diagnosis was long for all age groups.

All patients in the investigation were examined by the same physician and the same neuropsychologist. The patients were examined first by the physician in their own home.

The controls were selected from patients admitted to the surgical orthopaedic department for operations such as meniscus lesions, varicose veins, minor complaints of fingers and hands, etc. The controls had never suffered from infectious, or toxic or traumatic disorders of the CNS. Apart from their surgical admissions, they were healthy. They were recruited to the investigation after discharge from the surgical department, and from among suitable subjects it was possible to select a matched group of 39 persons. Their age range was between 25 and 55 years and, as can be seen from Table 4, they were matched as closely as possible with the MS patients for sex, age and social status.

Table 2. *Sex distribution of patient population.*

	Age groups (years)				
	25–35	*36–40*	*41–45*	*46–50*	*51–55*
MS population (n)					
Men	27	27	19	20	28
Women	33	35	32	33	31
MS patients examined (n)					
Men	10	11	8	9	12
Women	13	14	13	15	10
Proportion of MS patients examined (%)					
Men	37.0	40.7	42.1	45.0	42.9
Women	39.4	40.0	40.6	45.5	32.2

Table 3. *Sex distribution, mean age, Kurtzke disability status scale (KDSS), duration of disease from onset and diagnosis, Poser criteria*[11] *and social status, by age group.* Data are numbers of patients.

		Age groups (years)				
		25–35	*36–40*	*41–45*	*46–50*	*51–55*
Sex						
Men		10	11	8	9	12
Women		13	14	13	15	10
Age						
Mean (s.d.)		31.39 (3.12)	38.56 (1.42)	43.43 (1.60)	48.54 (1.14)	52.68 (1.29)
Duration of disease (years)						
1st symptom mean (s.d.)		8.39 (2.82)	10.36 (5.39)	17.67 (8.42)	17.17 (7.53)	16.64 (7.83)
Diagnosis mean (s.d.)		5.65 (3.27)	5.72 (4.03)	9.76 (6.36)	10.46 (4.71)	9.91 (5.71)
KDSS score						
1		6	1	1		2
2		5	2		3	1
3		2	10	8	7	9
4		2	6	3	7	5
5		1	3		2	
6		3	1	5	1	3
7		2	1	4	2	
8		1	1			2
9		1			2	
Poser criteria						
CDMS[a]	A1	20	22	19	22	19
	A2	1				
LSDMS[b]	B1	2	1	2	2	3
	B2		2	1		
Social groups						
1			1	1	1	
2		2	2	1		2
3		3	4	4	6	3
4		10	10	7	11	12
5		8	8	8	6	5

[a]CDMS = Clinical definite multiple sclerosis; [b]LSDMS = Laboratory-supported definite multiple sclerosis

Table 4. *Comparison of MS patients and controls*

	MS patients (age 42.8 years, s.d. 7.7)		*Controls (age 39.7 years, s.d. 8.3)*	
	Number	*Percent*	*Number*	*Percent*
Male	50	43.5	17	43.6
Female	65	56.5	22	56.4
Total	115			
Social status groups:				
I	3	2.6	1	2.6
II	7	6.1	2	5.1
III	20	17.4	7	17.9
IV	51	44.3	18	46.1
V	34	29.6	11	28.2

Table 5. *Neuropsychological test battery.*

WAIS test	*Attention and Perceptual Motor Speed Test*	*Memory tests*	*Screening test for latent aphasia*
1 Information	1 Trail Making Test parts A & B	1 Auditive Verbal Learning Test	1 The Token Test (short version)
2 Digit Span	2 The Symbol Digit Modalities Test	2 Story Recall	
3 Arithmetic		3 Recurring Figures Test	
4 Vocabulary		4 The Visual Gestalt Test	
5 Similarities			
6 Picture Arrangement			
7 Block Design			

Table 5 shows the test battery used. The first two memory tests measure verbal memory, the third and fourth measure visual memory. Analysis has shown that these four tests measure different forms of memory. This means that knowledge of a patient's performance in one test does not allow prediction of his/her performance in any of the others. From corresponding analyses we know that the two tests for attention and perceptual motor speed measure the same abilities. Both are included, since the Symbol Digit Modalities Test can be employed both orally and in the written form while the Trail Making Test is in written form. The oral form is naturally an advantage for MS patients. An explanation of how the tests are used is given with the results.

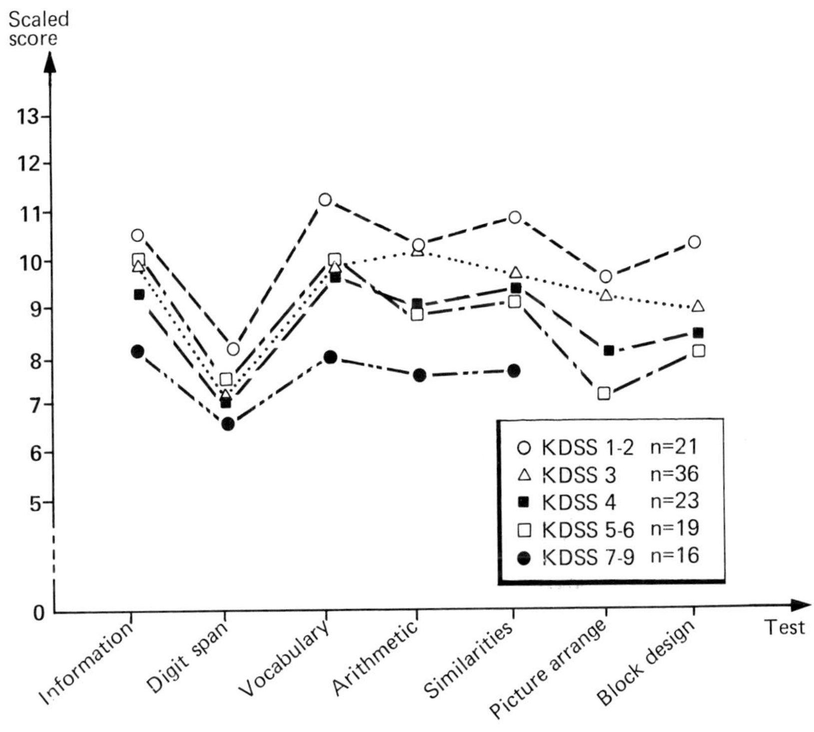

Fig. 1. *The WAIS-R Subtests* versus *Kurtzke Disability Status Scale (KDSS).*

Results

We have ensured that the results of all neuropsychological tests are independent of age for the MS group. It has therefore been possible to include all 115 patients and then to classify them according to the KDSS. As can be seen from the results, some of the KDSS groups have been combined to obtain a reasonable number of individuals in each. We have ensured suitable controls so that this combining of groups has not influenced the results.

The results of the intelligence tests were as follows. Comparison of the 39 controls with the 115 MS patients showed that there was no significant difference between them in two of the WAIS-R subtests, namely 'Information' and 'Vocabulary'. In all the other subtests the performance of the MS patients was significantly poorer ($P<0.05$).

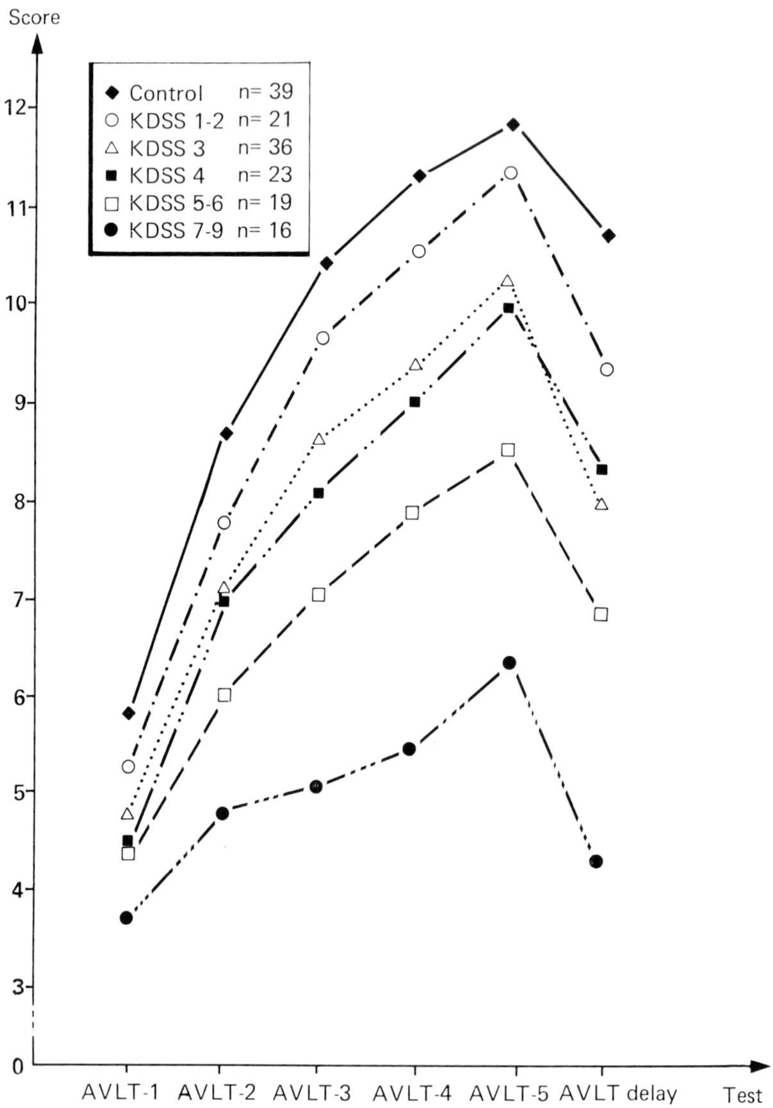

Fig. 2. *Auditive Verbal Learning Test (AVLT)* versus *Kurtzke Disability Status Scale Test (KDSS)*.

The mean values for each subtest in WAIS-R were calculated for each KDSS group (Fig. 1). There is a trend towards decline in mean value with increasing physical disability. The mean value for controls lies between KDSS 1–2 and KDSS 3. We found that the mean value for the KDSS group 7–9 was significantly lower than the control value. This means that intelligence impairment is seen in advanced MS as a consequence of the disease.

Figure 2 shows the Auditive Verbal Learning Test (AVLT), which measures short term memory, learning and delayed verbal memory. The procedure is that 15 words are read out and the subject repeats them in free recall, in all five times. After 15 minutes the patient is asked how many he remembers.

It is clearly apparent that performance became poorer with growing physical disability. The performance of patients with KDSS scores higher than 3 is significantly poorer than that of the controls ($P<0.01$). For the MS patients in KDSS groups 1–2 and 3, performance was significantly better than that of patients with high KDSS scores.

Figure 3 shows the results for story recall, which measures logical verbal memory. A story is read to the patient who must then repeat it word for word; if he is unable to do so, he is asked to recount it. The figure shows clearly that logical verbal memory declined with increasing physical disability. The performance of the control group was significantly better than that of the MS patients, whatever the KDSS group ($P<0.005$).

Figure 4 shows the results of the Recurring Figures Test, which measures non-verbal pattern recognition and short-term visual memory. The procedure is as follows. From a bank of 120 cards, each containing a line drawing of either a geometrical figure or an irregular nonsense figure, 20 designs are shown during presentation trials, and eight of these designs recur once during each recognition trial. There are five blocks of recognition trials, and the patient is tested for accurate recognition.

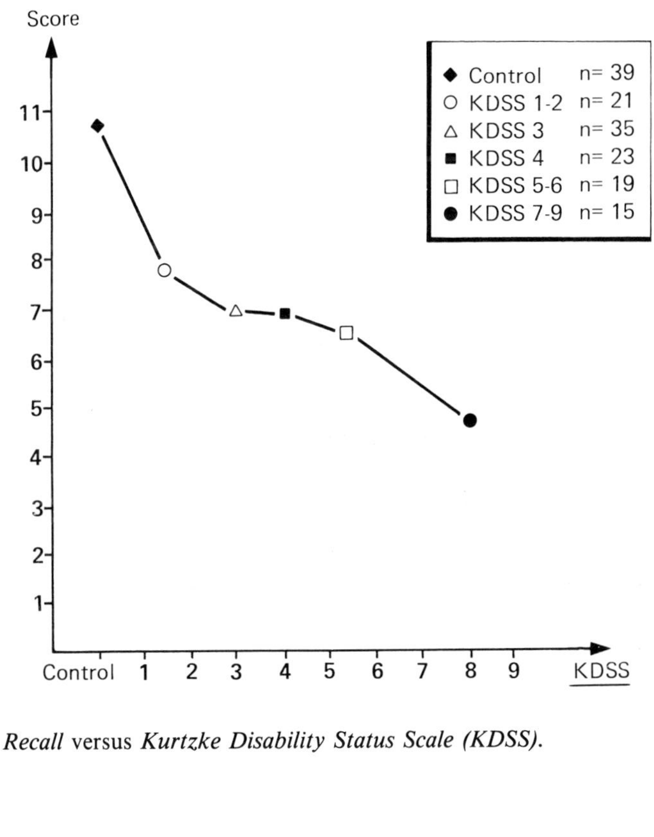

Fig. 3. *Story Recall* versus *Kurtzke Disability Status Scale (KDSS).*

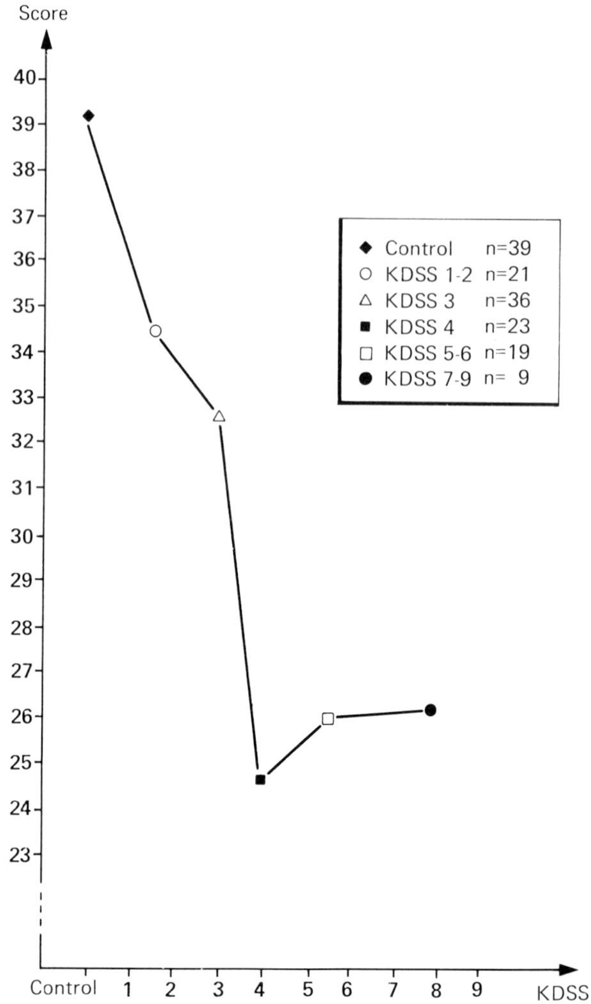

Fig. 4. *Recurring Figures Test* versus *Kurtzke Disability Status Scale (KDSS).*

Here again it can be seen that performance declined with increasing physical disability. Performance in the control group was significantly better than in MS patients with KDSS scores greater than 1–2 ($P<0.02$). For patients with KDSS scores greater than 3, there was no further decline in performance in this test, in spite of greater disability.

The results of the Visual Gestalt Test, which measures immediate recall, learning and delayed recall of logical visual information, are shown in Fig. 5. In this test four cards are used with drawings containing four geometrical figures. The patient looks at them for 10 seconds and must then draw them as well as he can. He draws them again from memory after 1 hour.

Patients in KDSS groups with scores higher than 3 performed significantly worse than controls on immediate recall and learning ability.

Figure 6 shows the tests of attention and perceptual motor speed. In the Trail Making test, part A, letters must be sorted out into alphabetical order. In part B, 1 must correspond

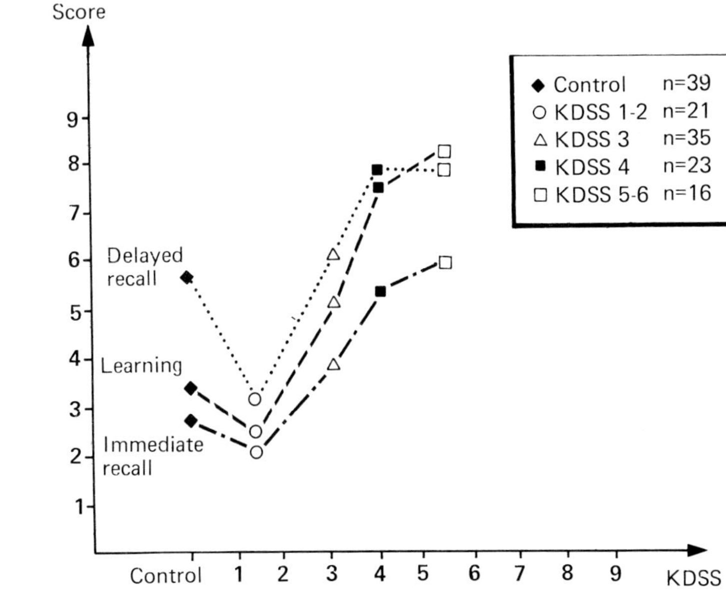

Fig. 5. *The Visual Gestalt Test* versus *Kurtzke Disability Status Scale (KDSS).*

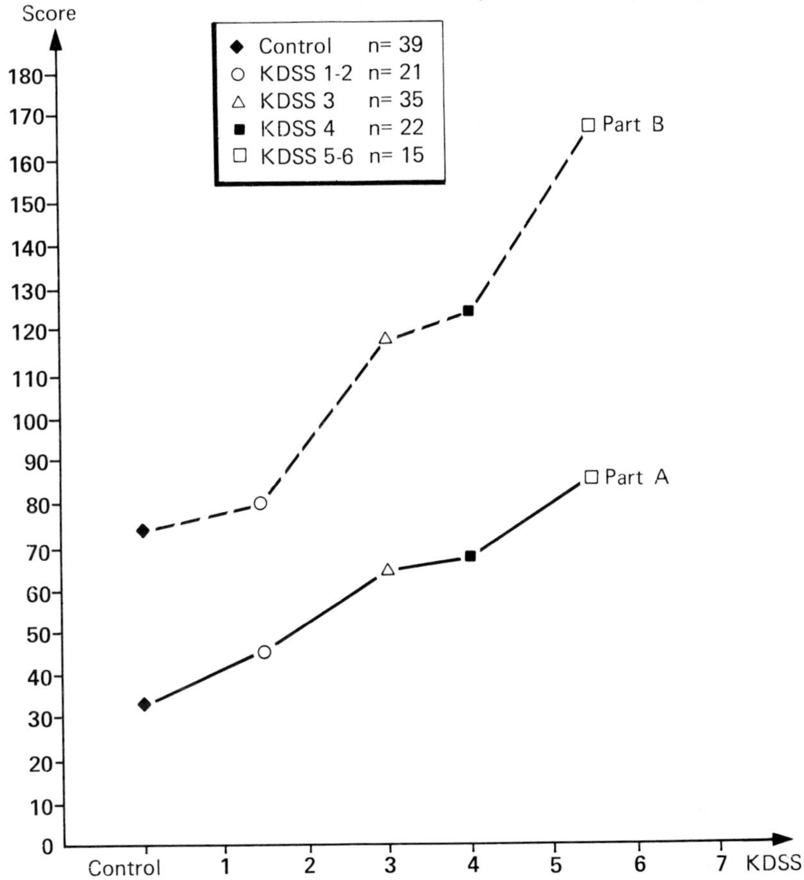

Fig. 6. *Trail Making* versus *Kurtzke Disability Status Test (KDSS).*

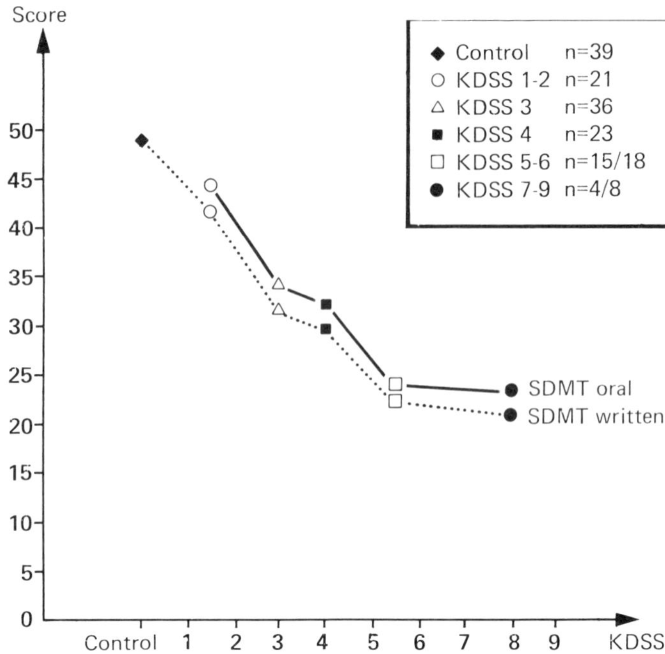

Fig. 7. *The Symbol Digit Modalities Test* versus *Kurtzke Disability Status Scale (KDSS).*

to a, 2 to b, etc. The time taken to carry out the test is recorded. The results in the MS patients became poorer with increasing physical disability, and the control group performed better than the patients, whatever their KDSS classification ($P < 0.005$).

In the Symbol Digit Modalities Test (SDMT), figures must be related to numbers, using a given code. The patient presents the solution to the test first in written form and then orally. The results of this test (Fig. 7) were in complete agreement with the results of the Trail Making test.

As mentioned in the introduction, deterioration has previously been interpreted as conditioned by decline in motor skills. If this were the case, the patient's performance in oral tests should be within the normal range, particularly when account is taken of the learning effect. This was not the case, and the implication is that deterioration is not the result of motor impairment but is due to a decline in mental abilities.

Conclusions

Our investigation covered 115 patients with definite MS, ranging in age from 25 to 55 years, and who were representative of MS patients admitted to the Neurological Department at Odense University Hospital between 1973 and 1985. They were compared with 39 healthy control persons from the same geographical region and matched for sex, age and social status.

Our findings are as follows: (1) the performance of MS patients in intelligence tests, memory tests and attention and perceptual motor speed tests was significantly worse than that of the controls; (2) impairment of intelligence occurred in severely disabled patients; (3) verbal memory declined in parallel with increased physical disability; (4) visual memory was severely impaired in patients whose KDSS classification was greater than 3; (5) attention and perceptual motor speed declined concurrently with increasing disability; and (6) this decline in performance was not conditioned by motor dysfunction but by a slowing down of general mental abilities. These findings can be expressed in a single sentence: cognitive impairment increases with increasing physical disability.

It is hardly necessary to stress that these findings apply to groups and therefore give no indication of the individual prognosis in terms of cognition. It is certainly possible for a severely handicapped MS patient to retain his cognitive function intact. At the same time, we know from other investigations that cognitive dysfunction tends to be overlooked, which is often why the therapist describes MS patients as difficult and prone to poor compliance. It is therefore important to realize that deterioration in the physical condition can go hand in hand with cognitive impairment.

Further investigation is needed to clarify the consequences of these cognitive deficits for the patients and their families to draw up guidelines for prevention or amelioration of this impairment.

Acknowledgements—This work was supported by Fonden for Scleroseramte på Fyn and the Danish Multiple Sclerosis Society. We wish to thank Jesper Boldsen, PhD, for assisting with the statistical analyses.

References

1 Kurtzke, J. F. (1983): Rating neurologic impairment in multiple sclerosis. *Neurology* **33**, 1444–1452.

2 Marsh, G. G. (1980): Disability and intellectual function in multiple sclerosis patients. *J. Nerv. Ment. Dis.* **168**, 758–762.

3 Heaton, R. K., Nelson, L. M., Thompson, D. S., Burks, J. S. & Franklin, J. S. (1985): Neuropsychological findings in relapsing-remitting chronic-progressive multiple sclerosis. *J. Consult. Clin. Psychol.* **53**, 103–110.

4 Lyon-Caen, O., Jouvent, R., Hauser, S., Chaunu, M. P., Benoit, N., Widlöcher, D. & Lhermitte, F. (1986): Cognitive function in recent onset demyelinating diseases. *Arch. Neurol.* **43**, 1138–1141.

5 Van den Burg, W., van Zomern, A. H., Minderhoud, J. M., Prange, A. J. A. & Meijer, N. S. A. (1987): Cognitive impairment in patients with multiple sclerosis and mild physical disability. *Arch. Neurol.* **44**, 494–501.

6 Grant, I., McDonald, W. I., Trimble, M. R., Schmit, E. & Reed, R. (1984): Deficient learning and memory in early and middle phases of multiple sclerosis. *J. Neurol. Neurosurg. Psychiatry* **47**, 250–255.

7 Ivnik, R. J. (1978): Neuropsychological test performance as a function of the duration of MS-related symptomatology. *J. Clin. Psychiatry* **39**, 304–312.

8 Ivnik, R. J. (1978): Neuropsychological stability in multiple sclerosis. *J. Consult. Clin. Psychol.* **46**, 913–923.

9 Beatty, P. A. & Grange, J. J. (1977): Neuropsychological aspects of multiple sclerosis. *J. Nerv. Ment. Dis.* **164**, 42–50.

10 Bertrando, P., Maffei, C. & Ghezzi, A. (1983): A study of neuropsychological alterations in multiple sclerosis. *Acta Psychiatry Belg.* **83**, 13–21.

11 Poser, C. M., Paty, D., Scheinberg, L., McDonald, W. I., Davis, F. A., Ebers, G. C., Johnson, K. P., Sibley, W. A., Silberberg, D. H. & Tourtellotte, W. W. (1983): New diagnostic criteria for multiple sclerosis: Guidelines for research protocols. *Ann. Neurol.* **13**, 227–231.

5

OBJECTIVE MEMORY TESTING IN MULTIPLE SCLEROSIS

Jill S. Fischer

Mellen Center for MS Treatment and Research, Cleveland Clinic Foundation, Cleveland, Ohio, USA

Summary

In order to characterize memory deficits and determine the need for objective memory testing in multiple sclerosis (MS), the Wechsler Memory Scale-Revised (WMS-R) and several subjective memory measures were administered to 45 patients with definite multiple sclerosis and 25 age-, sex-, and education-matched normal controls. As a group, MS patients performed significantly more poorly than normal controls on the five WMS-R summary scores ($P < 0.05$). Although patients' self-ratings of impairment were higher than those of controls ($P < 0.05$), greater perceived impairment was significantly associated with depression ($r = 0.43$), and not with impaired performance on objective testing (in all cases $r < 0.15$). Ratings by relatives, neurologists and a psychologist were somewhat more accurate, but correlations with objective memory performance were still modest (in all cases $r < -0.39$). Using cluster analysis, three subgroups of MS patients were identified on the basis of their performance on objective memory measures: the majority (56%) had intact attention but mild learning and long-term memory deficits; a smaller group (20%) had marked deficits in attention, learning and memory; the remainder (24%) were intact. The need for objective memory testing in MS and the utility of the WMS-R in routine memory assessment in MS are discussed.

Introduction

Memory complaints are relatively common among multiple sclerosis (MS) patients. In recent years, MS patients' memory deficits have been documented empirically as well. There is now consistent evidence that MS patients as a group are impaired in their learning and retention of both verbal and non-verbal material.[1-10] However, not all MS patients experience memory impairment. For example, Staples & Lincoln[9] reported that about

60 percent of their sample of patients with 'severe longstanding disability' showed some evidence of memory impairment. Rao and his colleagues[8] reported that, out of a group of patients with chronic/progressive MS, about 49 percent were mildly impaired while another 14 percent exhibited significant deficits in attention, learning, and long-term recall.

In clinical settings, however, objective memory testing is rarely part of a standard evaluation. Instead, decisions are often based on the patient's report of memory difficulties or on the impression of a neurologist or family member. This is problematic, though, because studies of neurological and psychiatric patients and of normal individuals have indicated that memory self-ratings often correlate poorly with objective measures of memory performance.[11,12,21–24] Furthermore, there is evidence to suggest that, when asked to judge overall cognitive impairment, neurologists make numerous false negative errors.[13] Until there has been systematic investigation of the relationship between subjective and objective assessments of memory impairment in MS, inferences based on clinical judgments or patients' reports must be suspect.

Unfortunately, the study of memory impairment in MS has been hampered somewhat by the lack of a uniform procedure for objective memory assessment; to date, investigators have used at least 20 different testing procedures to study memory impairment in MS. However, a recent revision and expansion of the Wechsler Memory Scale (WMS)[14] holds the promise of being an objective procedure that could systematize memory assessment in MS. The Wechsler Memory Scale-Revised (WMS-R)[15] has addressed many of the criticisms levelled at the original measure, incorporating three new non-verbal subtests, explicit scoring criteria, and a delayed recall condition for selected subtests.

The present study was undertaken to: (1) determine the utility of the WMS-R as an objective measure of memory impairment in MS; (2) investigate the relationship between subjective memory ratings and objective memory performance; and (3) examine the prevalence and characteristics of memory impairment in MS.

Methods

Two groups of subjects were tested: 45 MS patients (27 females, 18 males) with a mean age of 39.4 years (s.d. 8.3) and a mean of 14.2 years of education (s.d. 2.4), and 25 individuals (19 females, 6 males) without neurological or systemic illness who were matched to the MS group on age, sex, and education characteristics.

MS patients were drawn from those presenting to a comprehensive outpatient MS treatment and research centre for evaluation. They fulfilled Poser criteria[16] for 'clinically-definite' or 'laboratory-supported definite' MS and had no other neurological or systemic diseases that might influence cognitive functioning, nor any history of alcohol or other drug abuse. They had to have sufficient vision and hand strength/coordination to perform the non-verbal memory tasks.

The MS patients in this study had carried a diagnosis of MS for a mean of 4.9 years (s.d. 4.8), although they had had symptoms for a mean of 9.5 years (s.d. 6.5). Despite the aforementioned restrictions, the MS group had a broad range of physical disability, ranging from 0.0 to 8.0 on the Kurtzke Expanded Disability Status Scale (EDSS)[17], with a mean of 4.0 (s.d. 2.0). Seventeen patients (38%) were classified as having relapsing/remitting MS, 18 (40%) as relapsing/progressive, and 10 (22%) as chronic/progressive. Twenty-nine (67%) were considered by a neurologist to have active disease at the time of testing. Nine (20%) were taking medication likely to have sedative-hypnotic effects; an additional 19 (42%) were taking medication with other CNS effects (eg β-blockers and anticholinergics).

Normal controls (NC) were recruited through advertisements directed at Cleveland Clinic employees and from family members and friends of MS patients. They were screened to rule out neurological and systemic diseases thought to affect cognitive functioning. None of the NC group was taking medications with sedative-hypnotic effects, but seven (28%) were taking medications with other CNS effects.

Prior to objective memory testing, all subjects completed a subjective memory measure (Patient's Assessment of Own Functioning Inventory, PAF)[11] and the Beck Depression Inventory (BDI)[18] prior to administration of the WMS-R. In addition, a friend or relative completed two subjective memory measures, the Relative's Assessment of Patient's Functioning Inventory (RAF)[11] and the Memory Rating Form (MRF), an unpublished measure developed by The Psychological Corporation. Finally, a neurologist and a psychologist, each of whom had evaluated the patient clinically, made independent ratings of the patient's memory impairment on a 0 (none) to 3 (severe) scale.

The WMS-R was used in all subjects to assess objective memory performance. This consists of 10 subtests, four of which are repeated after a 30 minute delay. Five indices can be computed, each of which is adjusted for age and standardized to a mean of 100 and a standard deviation of 15. These are Attention-Concentration Index (ACI), General Memory Index (GMI), Verbal Memory Index (VBMI), Visual Memory Index (VSMI), and Delayed Recall Index (DRI). The ACI can be considered a measure of attention/short-term memory; the GMI a mixture of short-term memory, learning, and long-term memory; and the DRI a pure measure of long-term memory. The VBMI and the VSMI are essentially subsets of the GMI.

Results

As expected, the MS group performed more poorly on the WMS-R than did matched controls (Table 1). A multivariate analysis of variance (MANOVA) of the three non-redundant indices (ACI, GMI, and DRI) indicated that the overall group difference was statistically significant ($F_{3,66}=7.26$, $P<0.001$), as were group differences on each of the five indices analysed independently (in all cases $P<0.05$). As Table 1 shows, fully 40% of the MS group scored more than 2 s.d. below the control mean on the DRI; this suggests that significant long-term memory impairment occurs in MS at a rate 16 times that of the normal population.

Note also that scores of the MS group were technically within normal limits on all five indices and that scores of the NC group were consistently above the expected mean of 100;

Table 1. *WMS-R performance by group.*

	NC Group[a]		*MS Group*[b]			
Index	*Mean*	*s.d.*	*Mean*	*s.d.*	*% Impaired*[c]	*F*
Attention–Concentration (ACI)	105.68	10.77	96.78	13.25	22.2	8.25*
General Memory (GMI)	109.60	11.48	96.02	17.30	28.9	12.33‡
Verbal Memory (VBMI)	108.20	10.56	98.76	14.24	22.2	8.40*
Visual Memory (VSMI)	105.64	12.24	92.42	17.71	20.0	10.98†
Delayed Recall (DRI)	108.32	11.63	91.73	16.55	40.0	19.66‡

[a]n = 25; [b]n = 45; [c]Percent scoring more than 2 s.d. below the mean of the NC group. NC = normal controls; MS = multiple sclerosis.
*$P<0.005$; †$P<0.002$; ‡$P<0.001$.

this is attributable to the fact that subjects in this study were more educated than the normative group for the WMS-R, and hence scored better. It also suggests that education be taken into account when interpreting the performance of individual patients on this and other memory measures.

At first glance, results from the subjective memory measures are generally consistent with WMS-R results. For example, the PAF-Memory subscale scores of MS patients as a group indicated significantly greater perceived impairment (mean 13.49) than those of normal controls (mean 9.28) ($F1,68 = 4.26$, $P < 0.05$). Similarly, relatives' ratings of MS patients' memory impairment were significantly higher (mean 24.12) than those of normal controls (mean 20.04) on the MRF ($F1,64 = 4.48$, $P < 0.05$), although they did not differ significantly on the RAF-Memory subscale (means 11.47 and 10.63, respectively).

However, most of the correlations between MS patients' subjective and objective memory measures were disappointingly low (see Table 2). Perhaps most striking is how little relationship patients' self-ratings bore to their objective memory performance. In fact, patients' self-ratings correlated more highly with depression, as assessed by the BDI ($r = 0.43$), than they did with any of the WMS-R indexes. Ratings by others (neurologists, psychologist, and relatives) correlated more highly with WMS-R performance than did the patient's own ratings; however, although several of the correlations between others' ratings and WMS-R indices were statistically significant, subjective estimates of memory impairment accounted for at most 15% of the variance in patients' WMS-R performance.

In an effort to increase the predictive validity of subjective ratings, a consensus memory impairment rating was constructed from the subjective ratings of the neurologists, psychologist, and relatives. MS patients who were adjudged impaired by two of the three raters were assigned to an 'impaired' group, while others were placed in the 'intact' group; 55 percent of the MS group were judged to be impaired. (To construct this index, the neurologists' and psychologist's ratings were each collapsed into two categories [0 = intact and 1 = impaired]; relatives' MRF scores were also dichotomized [$\leqslant 28$ = intact and > 28 = impaired].)

As expected, correlations between the consensus rating and WMS-R index scores were generally stronger than those between individual subjective ratings and objective

Table 2. *Correlations between subjective and objective memory measures—MS group.*

Index	*Rater*					
	Patient[a]	*Neurologist*	*Psychologist*	*Relative MRF*[b]	*Relative RAF-M*[c]	*Consensus rating*
Attention–Concentration (ACI)	0.02	−0.07	−0.03	−0.09	0.09	0.00
General Memory (GMI)	0.03	−0.28*	−0.32*	−0.34*	−0.29*	$-0.49^{\ddagger}$
Verbal Memory (VBMI)	0.02	−0.16	−0.28*	$-0.36^{\dagger}$	−0.31*	$-0.46^{\ddagger}$
Visual Memory (VSMI)	0.00	$-0.36^{\dagger}$	−0.30*	−0.23	−0.19	$-0.40^{\dagger}$
Delayed Recall (DRI)	0.14	$-0.39^{\dagger}$	−0.29*	−0.11	−0.25	$-0.41^{\dagger}$

Note: On all subjective measures, higher scores are associated with greater impairment, so negative correlations indicate greater concordance between subjective and objective measures.
[a]Patient's Assessment of Own Functioning Inventory-Memory subscale; [b]Memory Rating Form; [c]Relative's Assessment of Patient's Functioning Inventory-Memory subscale.
$*P < 0.05$; $^{\dagger}P < 0.01$; $^{\ddagger}P < 0.001$.

performance (see Table 2). However, even the consensus rating accounted for less than 25 percent of the variance in WMS-R index scores. Furthermore, there was a great deal of overlap in WMS-R index scores of the adjudged 'intact' and 'impaired' groups. For example, GMI scores of patients who were rated intact ranged from 65–128, while those of patients rated to be impaired were 63–115. Similarly, DRI scores of adjudged 'intact' patients ranged from 60 to 128, virtually identical to the range of 57–113 for patients judged to be impaired. Thus subjective impressions of memory impairment are of little value in predicting the performance of individual patients on objective memory measures.

The final purpose of this study was to examine the characteristics of memory impairment in MS. One approach is to use cluster analysis to identify relatively homogeneous subgroups based on their patterns of performance on key WMS-R indices. Because performance on memory measures is frequently related to demographic variables, scores on the three non-overlapping WMS-R indices (ACI, GMI, and DRI) were first regressed with age, sex, and education; then, standardized residual scores on these indices were submitted to a hierarchical cluster analysis, using the average linkage between groups method.[19]

The three cluster solution optimized group size and group differences. Table 3 presents descriptive statistics for these three clusters on each of the five WMS-R indexes. Over half of the MS group (56%) fell into a cluster with intact attention and mild impairment in learning, short-term memory, and long-term memory (Cluster 1). Another subgroup (20%) not only had moderate attentional deficits but also substantial learning and memory deficits (Cluster 3). Finally, the performance of another cluster of comparable size (Cluster 2) was intact; in fact, patients in this cluster outperformed matched controls in many respects.

Although the MS group as a whole did not exhibit differential impairment on verbal and non-verbal measures (relative to the NC group), one subgroup of MS patients, Cluster 3, appeared to be more impaired than the other two clusters on the non-verbal measures of the GMI. To investigate this statistically, VBMI and VSMI scores for the three clusters were compared using a mixed model ANOVA. The main effect for Cluster was statistically significant ($F_{2,42}=78.42$, $P<0.001$), as was the main effect for Modality ($F_{1,42}=16.52$, $P<0.001$). The Cluster × Modality interaction was also significant ($F_{2,42}=4.17$, $P<0.025$), attesting to the relatively greater visual memory impairment of Cluster 3.

In order to characterize the performance of the three clusters further, WMS-R subtest scores were converted to T-scores based on the means and standard deviations of the NC group. Mean T-scores for the three clusters on each of the subtests are depicted graphically in Fig. 1.

Table 3. *Descriptive statistics for WMS-R Index scores of MS patients by cluster.*

	Cluster 1[a]		*Cluster 2*[b]		*Cluster 3*[c]	
Index	*Mean*	*s.d.*	*Mean*	*s.d.*	*Mean*	*s.d.*
Attention–Concentration (ACI)	99.00	10.04	103.82	14.96	82.00	7.33
General Memory (GMI)	93.84	7.25	119.36	8.27	73.56	8.44
Verbal Memory (VBMI)	95.92	8.45	117.36	8.69	83.88	7.56
Visual Memory (VSMI)	93.80	9.50	110.00	13.37	67.11	8.84
Delayed Recall (DRI)	89.08	7.76	113.64	10.32	72.33	9.35

[a]n = 25; [b]n = 11; [c]n = 9.

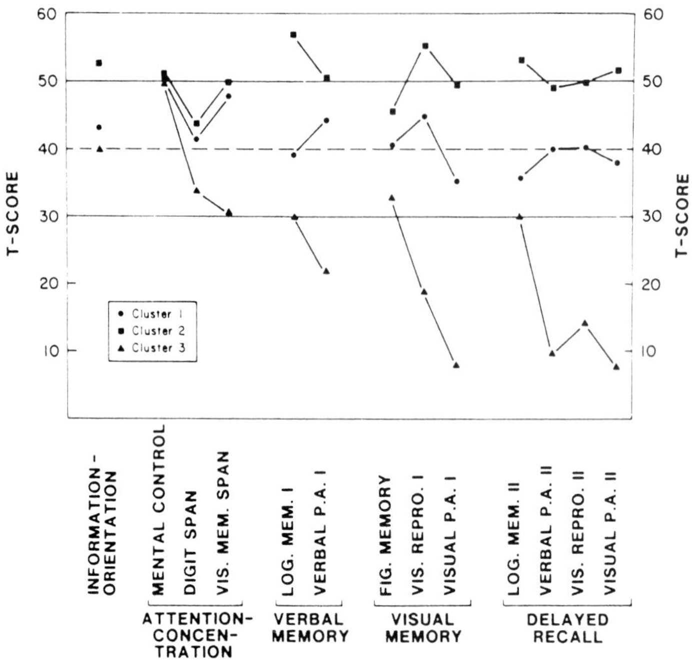

Fig. 1. *T-scores of MS clusters on WMS-R subtests.*

It is immediately evident that there are striking differences across clusters both in the level and in the pattern of performance across a number of subtests. Of the ACI subtests, the memory span subtests appeared to be the most sensitive to differences among the clusters. Although the three clusters performed comparably on Mental Control, patients in Cluster 3 exhibited significantly greater difficulty than those in either Clusters 1 or 2 on both Digit Span subtests, especially Digits Backward, and Visual Memory Span (in all cases $P<0.05$).

All three clusters can be differentiated on the basis of their level and pattern of performance on the GMI subtests. Looking first at Verbal Memory subtests, all three clusters differed significantly from each other on Logical Memory I ($P<0.01$), while Cluster 3 differed significantly from Clusters 1 and 2 (which did not differ significantly from each other) on Verbal Paired Associates I ($P<0.001$). Both Clusters 2 and 3 performed relatively more poorly on Verbal Paired Associates I than on Logical Memory I, whereas Cluster 1 showed the opposite pattern of performance.

All three clusters also differed significantly from each other on two of the three Visual Memory subtests, Visual Reproduction I and Visual Paired Associates I (in all cases $P<0.05$). There were only minor differences among the clusters in Figural Memory performance, however, suggesting that recognition tasks may be less sensitive than recall tasks in differentiating subgroups of MS patients. The three clusters also differed in their patterns of performance on the Visual Memory measures: Clusters 1 and 2 both exhibited an 'inverted V' pattern, with their best performance on Visual Reproduction I, whereas the best performance for Cluster 3 was on Figural Memory.

Finally, the three clusters can also be differentiated on the basis of their performance on DRI subtests. Again, Clusters 1 and 2 showed relatively similar patterns of performance, while Cluster 3 exhibited a different, more variable pattern of subtest performance. On Logical Memory II, the differences between the performance of Cluster 2 and those of Clusters 1 and 3 were statistically significant (in all cases $P<0.001$), but Clusters 1 and 3 did not differ significantly from each other. In contrast, on Verbal Paired Associates II and on Visual Paired Associates II, Cluster 3 performed significantly worse than Clusters 1 and 2 (in all cases $P<0.05$), which did not differ from each other. Finally, on Visual Reproduction II, all three clusters differed significantly from each other (in all cases $P<0.005$).

In order to investigate learning across clusters, mean number of items recalled on each trial of the two multitrial learning subtests (Verbal Paired Associates I and Visual Paired Associates I) was computed for each cluster. These learning curves, along with Delayed Recall performance (Hard Verbal Paired Associates II and Visual Paired Associates II) are presented graphically in Fig. 2. (Only Hard Verbal Paired Associates were analysed because Easy Associates failed to discriminate between the MS and control groups).

The clusters differed significantly in their performance on both Hard Verbal Paired Associates I (multivariate $F_{2,42}=18.21$, $P<0.001$) and Visual Paired Associates I (multivariate $F_{2,42}=15.49$, $P<0.001$). Although performance improved significantly across trials on both Hard Verbal Paired Associates I (multivariate $F_{5,38}=21.73$, $P<0.001$) and Visual Paired Associates I (multivariate $F_{5,38}=15.16$, $P<0.001$), the clusters learned Hard

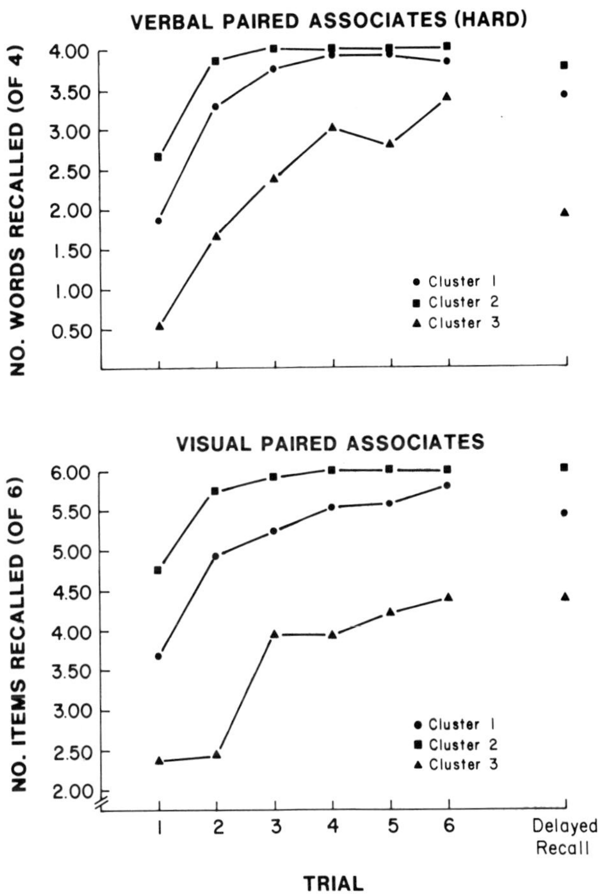

Fig. 2. *Performance of MS clusters across trials on WMS-R Paired Associates subtests.*

Verbal Associates I at significantly different rates (multivariate $F_{10,76}=2.15$, $P<0.05$). Although the learning curves of Clusters 1 and 2 were similar to that of the NC group and not statistically different from each other, the performance of Cluster 3 differed significantly from that of Clusters 1 and 2 on each of the first five trials (in all cases $P<0.001$); in other words, Cluster 3 started at a significant disadvantage and took six trials to 'catch up' to the other two. (On Visual Paired Associates I, the Cluster × Trials interaction did not achieve statistical significance, but the general pattern of results was the same).

Thus results of the cluster analysis suggest that there may be two subtypes of memory impairment in MS. The majority of memory-impaired MS patients show a pattern of performance similar to that of intact patients, but differ in their overall level of performance on learning and memory measures. A smaller subgroup of memory-impaired patients differs not only in the overall level but also in the pattern of their performance.

Finally, demographic and disease-related characteristics of the three clusters were examined in order to determine if extent and pattern of memory impairment could be predicted on the basis of any of these factors. There were no demographic differences across clusters, given that standardized residual scores (ie, scores from which the effects of age, sex, and education had been partialled out) had been used in constructing the clusters. More surprising was the fact that overall differences across clusters in disease duration, disease course, disease activity, and degree of physical impairment (Kurtzke EDSS) were also not statistically significant. The most impaired cluster (Cluster 3) did have a higher proportion (67%) of patients with relapsing-progressive disease, whereas Cluster 2 (the 'intact' cluster) was comprised primarily of individuals with relapsing-remitting disease (64%), however. Finally, the clusters did not differ significantly in terms of medication status (ie, proportion taking sedative-hypnotics or medications with other CNS effects), nor could differences in level of depression explain differences in WMS-R performance across the clusters. Thus there are few patient variables that can be used to guide clinicians' judgments about the memory functioning of individual patients.

Discussion

As expected, MS patients as a group performed significantly more poorly than a matched normal control group on the WMS-R, demonstrating the sensitivity of the WMS-R to memory deficits in MS. Furthermore, subgroups of MS patients with differing levels and patterns of memory impairment could be identified on the basis of their WMS-R performance, suggesting that the WMS-R may be useful in objectively assessing the memory functioning of individual patients.

Several indicators should be particularly helpful in the assessment of learning and memory deficits associated with MS. For example, numerous investigators have documented impaired learning in MS patients using other measures.[1,3–6,8–10] The relatively brief Verbal Paired Associates I (primarily Hard Verbal Paired Associates I) and Visual Paired Associates I subtests did a surprisingly good job of identifying MS patients with significant learning impairment. However, if one wants to differentiate those with mildly impaired learning from those whose learning is intact, a test explicitly designed to analyse learning strategies and retention over time, such as the California Verbal Learning Test (CVLT),[20] should be used. Second, Logical Memory I and Visual Reproduction I, as well as the proportion of information from these two subtests retained after a delay, should be useful in discriminating among patients with differing levels of memory impairment. The WMS-R also enables one to analyse differential performance on matched verbal and visual measures, the VBMI and the VSMI; the results of this study suggest that relatively poorer visual memory may be most characteristic of MS patients with global attentional and memory deficits. Finally, the DRI appears to be sensitive to the deficits in long-term recall frequently described by previous investigators.[2–4,6–10]

Thus, the WMS-R represents a significant advance in the measurement of attention, learning, and memory, one that should be useful and relatively efficient in monitoring these functions in MS patients over time. Norms based on education as well as age would be useful, however, to ensure accurate interpretation of the test results of individual patients.

Consistent with research using other populations,[11,12,21–23] subjective estimates of memory functioning were only modestly related to objective memory performance. Although MS patients often complain about memory impairment, results of the present study suggest that these complaints may be indicative of depression, rather than actual memory impairment. Ratings by others were more accurate than those of MS patients in predicting memory impairment, but even professionals were unable to predict a patient's memory functioning with any degree of accuracy that would be clinically useful.

The overall proportion of patients judged to be memory impaired was somewhat higher in this study than in that reported by Peyser and her colleagues.[13] It may well be that health care professionals have become more aware of the prevalence of cognitive impairment in MS since 1980, although the results of the present study suggests that their subjective impressions have not become any more accurate. Relying on the consensus of two or three raters improves the accuracy of subjective ratings to some extent, but even the consensus memory impairment rating is highly inaccurate in the case of individual patients. These findings call into question the standard practice of relying on subjective impressions of an individual's cognitive status and underscore the need to perform at least a brief neuropsychological evaluation routinely in the examination of MS patients.

One caveat about interpreting these results is in order. One could argue that the reason for the poor correlations between subjective ratings and objective performance is that raters are making estimates of 'everyday' memory functioning, whereas objective tests tap learning and memory in an artificial context. However, the few studies using tasks bearing a greater resemblance to everyday activities, such as remembering details from a recently-viewed film,[24] have also reported poor correlations between performance on these tasks and subjective ratings. Therefore, at present it is most reasonable to conclude that, under most conditions, subjective impressions of memory functioning are imprecise and need to be verified with objective memory assessment.

Which MS patients are likely to experience memory impairment? In this study, three subgroups of patients with different levels and patterns of WMS-R performance were identified. Approximately one in four patients (24%) was intact; WMS-R performance of these patients was not discriminable in any respect from that of a group of matched normal controls. About half (56%) exhibited mild selective impairment; for these patients, attention and short-term memory were intact, while learning and retention of new material was impaired. Although these two subgroups differed in their overall levels of performance, their patterns of performance across WMS-R subtests were generally similar. The remainder of the MS group (20%) was globally impaired; not only did they have significant attentional/short-term memory deficits, but they also had marked difficulty learning and retaining new information, particularly visual material.

The results of the cluster analysis in the present study essentially confirm those of Rao *et al.*,[8] who studied patients with chronic/progressive MS. They also derived three clusters of patients on the basis of their performance on several WMS subtests and other memory measures; proportions of patients in each of Rao *et al.*'s clusters differ from those in the present study due to differences in the samples studied and the measures used, but the patterns of performance of the clusters are much the same.

Unfortunately, the results of the present study and others suggest that degree of memory impairment in MS is not predictable on the basis of disease duration or disability,[1,3,7,8,10] nor is it a simple function of medication status or depression.[1,3,4,8,10] One intriguing finding in the present study is that the most impaired subgroup comprised a disproportionate number of patients with relapsing/progressive disease. Although previous investigators[4] have reported that patients with chronic/progressive MS are more likely than those with relapsing/remitting disease to exhibit cognitive impairment on a variety of measures, other researchers have not included relapsing/progressive MS in their classification scheme. The present study suggests that patients with relapsing/progressive disease may be prone to a more global dementia, so it would be useful to analyse the performance of these patients separately in the future.

One must be cautious, however, about interpreting the results of the cluster analysis in this study, as one should be about interpreting the results of any statistical analysis done on empirical rather than theoretical grounds. One could argue that, rather than identifying patients with distinct patterns of memory impairment (or lack of impairment), the cluster analysis merely identified groups of individuals who varied in terms of their initial level of memory functioning (high/average/low). Two factors make this unlikely: (1) the effects of education and other demographic factors on the WMS-R index scores were controlled prior to submitting them to cluster analysis; and (2) no subjects in the matched control group achieved WMS-R scores as low as those of subjects in Cluster 3. What this study cannot address, however, is whether all (or most) MS patients undergo a progressive decline in memory functioning, so that the cluster analysis has merely identified patients at different points on a continuum, or whether there are distinct patterns of memory impairment in MS. It remains for future investigators to track the course of memory impairment in MS over time, to determine the neuroanatomical correlates of different patterns of memory deficits, and to assess the impact of these deficits on the everyday functioning of MS patients and their families.

Acknowledgments—This research was funded in part by The Psychological Corporation, the Cleveland Clinic Foundation, and the Mellen Foundation. I could not have completed this work without assistance from Tony Breuer, Jack Conomy, Hershel Goren, and Rick Rudick in establishing the certainty of diagnosis and completing neurological ratings on the MS patients, and from Kathy Kawczak in testing subjects and coding data. Discussions with Gordon Chelune, Steve Rao, and Dave Rodgers were also helpful in stimulating my thinking about data analytic procedures and measurement issues. Portions of this paper were also presented at the Annual Meeting of the American Psychological Association, New York City, in August, 1987, and portions were reported in an article entitled 'Using the Wechsler Memory Scale-Revised to Detect and Characterize Memory Deficits in Multiple Sclerosis', which appeared in *The Clinical Neuropsychologist*, Vol 2, No 2 (1988).

References

1 Beatty, P. A. & Gange, J. J. (1977): Neuropsychological aspects of multiple sclerosis. *J. Nerv. Ment. Dis.* **164**, 42–50.

2 Caine, E. D., Bamford, K. A., Schiffer, R. B., Shoulson, I. & Levy, S. (1986): A controlled neuropsychological comparison of Huntington's disease and multiple sclerosis. *Arch. Neurol.* **43**, 249–254.

3 Grant, I., McDonald, W. I., Trimble, M. R., Smith, E. & Reed, R. (1984): Deficient learning and memory in early and middle phases of multiple sclerosis. *J. Neurol. Neurosurg. Psychiatry* **47**, 250–255.

4 Heaton, R. K., Nelson, L. M., Thompson, D. S., Burks, J. S. & Franklin, G. M. (1985): Neuropsychological findings in relapsing-remitting and chronic-progressive multiple sclerosis. *J. Consult. Clin. Psychol.* **53**, 103–110.

5 Huber, S. J., Paulson, G. W., Shuttleworth, E. C., Chakeres, D., Clapp, L. E., Pakalnis, A., Weiss, K. & Rammohan, K. (1987): Magnetic resonance imaging correlates of dementia in multiple sclerosis. *Arch. Neurol.* **44**, 732–736.

6 Jambor, K. L. (1969): Cognitive functioning in multiple sclerosis. *Br. J. Psychiatry* **115**, 765–775.
7 Lyon-Caen, O., Jouvent, R., Hauser, S., Chaunu, M-P., Benoit, N., Widlocher, D. & Lhermitte, F. (1986): Cognitive function in recent-onset demyelinating diseases. *Arch. Neurol.* **43**, 1138–1141.
8 Rao, S. M., Hammeke, T. A., McQuillen, M. P., Khatri, B. O. & Lloyd, D. (1984): Memory disturbance in chronic progressive multiple sclerosis. *Arch. Neurol.* **41**, 625–631.
9 Staples, D. & Lincoln, N. B. (1979): Intellectual impairment in multiple sclerosis and its relation to functional abilities. *Rheum. Rehab.* **18**, 153–160.
10 van den Burg, W., van Zomeren, A. H., Minderhoud, J. M., Prange, A. J. A. & Meijer, N. S. A. (1987): Cognitive impairment in patients with multiple sclerosis and mild physical disability. *Arch. Neurol.* **44**, 494–501.
11 Chelune, G. J., Heaton, R. K. & Lehman, R. A. W. (1986): Neuropsychological and personality correlates of patients' complaints of disability. In *Advances in clinical neuropsychology, Vol. 3*, ed G. Goldstein & R. E. Tarter, pp 95–126. New York: Plenum.
12 Williams, J. M., Little, M. M., Scates, S. & Blockman, N. (1987): Memory complaints and abilities among older adults. *J. Consult. Clin. Psychol.* **55**, 595–598.
13 Peyser, J., Edwards, K. R., Poser, C. & Filskov, S. (1980): Cognitive function in patients with multiple sclerosis. *Arch. Neurol.* **37**, 577–579.
14 Wechsler, D. (1945): A standardized memory scale for clinical use. *J. Psychol.* **19**, 87–95.
15 Wechsler, D. (1987): *WMS-R: Wechsler Memory Scale-Revised manual.* San Antonio: The Psychological Corporation.
16 Poser, C., Paty, D., Scheinberg, L., McDonald, W. I., Davis, F. A., Ebers, G. C., Johnson, K. P., Sibley, W. A., Silberberg, D. H. & Tourtellotte, W. W. (1983): New diagnostic criteria for multiple sclerosis: Guidelines for research protocols. *Ann. Neurol.* **13**, 227–231.
17 Kurtzke, J. F. (1983): Rating neurologic impairment in multiple sclerosis: An expanded disability status scale (EDSS). *Neurology* **33**, 1444–1452.
18 Beck, A. T., Ward, C. H., Mendelson, M., Mock, J. & Erbaugh, J. (1961): An inventory for measuring depression. *Arch. Gen. Psychiatry* **4**, 561–571.
19 Norusis, M. J. (1983): *SPSS^X advanced statistics guide.* New York: McGraw-Hill.
20 Delis, D. C., Kramer, J. H., Kaplan, E. & Ober, B. A. (1987): *CVLT: California Verbal Learning Test manual.* San Antonio: The Psychological Corporation.
21 Herrmann, D. J. (1982): Know thy memory: The use of questionnaires to assess and study memory. *Psychol. Bull.* **92**, 434–452.
22 Larrabee, G. J. & Levin, H. S. (1986): Memory self-ratings and objective test performance in a normal elderly sample. *J. Clin. Exp. Neuropsychol.* **8**, 275–284.
23 Sunderland, A., Harris, J. E. & Baddeley, A. D. (1983): Do laboratory tests predict everyday memory? A neuropsychological study. *J. Verb. Lrng. Verb. Beh.* **22**, 341–357.
24 Morris, P. E. (1984): The validity of subjective reports on memory. In *Everyday memory, actions, and absent-mindedness*, ed J. E. Harris & P. E. Morris, pp 153–172. London: Academic Press.

III

COGNITION, MAGNETIC RESONANCE IMAGING AND CEREBRAL BLOOD FLOW

6

MAGNETIC RESONANCE IMAGING STUDIES IN MULTIPLE SCLEROSIS

D. W. Paty

Division of Neurology, University of British Columbia, Vancouver, BC, Canada

Summary

Magnetic Resonance Imaging (MRI) has opened a window on the brain that is helping in the understanding of the evolution of the MS process. It is the most sensitive method for showing dissemination of lesions in space. The extent of the lesions can be measured in order to determine extent of disease. Frequent MRI examinations also show that disease activity is much greater than would be suspected by clinical evaluation alone. Through the systematic application of MRI techniques we will probably understand the evolution of the MS process much better in the future.

Introduction

The ability of magnetic resonance imaging (MRI) to visualize the lesions of multiple sclerosis (MS) has created a considerable amount of excitement in the MS community. The most immediate impact of MRI on MS has been in increasing the accuracy of diagnosis. However, in the long-term, the major impact of MRI is likely to be in the area of disease monitoring. MRI can very precisely identify the areas of abnormality in MS, and then allow one to follow the evolution of those lesions over time. This ability to reveal the evolution of the pathological process is going to help considerably in the understanding of the pathogenesis of MS and the correlation between lesions and symptoms.

Pathological correlation studies[1] are validating the sensitivity and specificity of the technique, and it is clear that MRI studies will help answer the question of whether the clinical nature of MS as a phasic disorder reflects the actual nature of the pathology. Is MS a truly phasic process, or is there continuous evolution of pathology with only intermittent symptoms reflecting both the location and the intrinsic qualities of the lesions?

The most specific and characteristic pathological change in MS is demyelination. Specific demyelination occurs when there is loss of the myelin sheath with preservation of axons. In addition to demyelination, we also know that in acute lesions of MS, though pathological experience is generally limited, inflammation can be quite intense.[2] The inflammation in MS is marked by the presence of immunoglobulins, lymphocytes and plasma cells. Macrophages are also present, and are active in the process of damage to myelin. The immunoglobulins in the cerebrospinal fluid (CSF) are usually present in a pattern referred to as oligoclonal banding (OB) which is very useful in diagnosis. OB is a necessary component to satisfy the diagnostic criteria for laboratory-supported definite multiple sclerosis.[3] The very first event in the development of the acute MS lesion may be breakdown in the blood-brain barrier (BBB).[4] The enhanced CT scan can demonstrate BBB disruption, but CSF albumin, usually used as a marker of this process, is not markedly elevated in MS. In the future, MRI will be able to distinguish between lesions that are primarily inflammatory as opposed to those that are demyelinating and/or gliotic in nature. Gadolineum can be used as a marker of BBB disruption allowing MRI not only to measure the number and extent of lesions but also to identify those lesions that are presumably acute.

Gliosis develops in the later stages of lesion evolution in MS. A gliotic scar is produced by the proliferation of astrocytes, probably during the subacute phase of lesion development. Fog & Linnemann[5] have proposed that the chronic evolving clinical deficit in MS may be, in part, due to gliosis.

There have been a number of imaging methods used in the study of MS. Radionuclide brain scanning was the first technique used, but it was found to be very insensitive to the MS lesions.[6] Positron emission tomography (PET) has also been found to be abnormal in some patients with MS, but it is also very insensitive to MS lesions.[7] In addition, the resolution of PET is not great enough to identify most individual MS lesions.

Computerized X-ray tomography (CT) studies have shown that 36 percent of MS patients have low density lesions in their periventricular white matter.[8] Subsequent studies using contrast enhancement, particularly using high volume delayed (HVD) contrast, have shown that multiple enhancing lesions are not at all unusual.[9] Multiple enhancing lesions in the white matter are characteristic of MS, particularly during acute relapse. These lesions are so characteristic that they can be used to satisfy the criteria for dissemination in space.[3] The enhancing lesions can resolve very quickly and are susceptible to the effects of corticosteroids. In addition to showing low density and enhancing lesions on CT, many patients with long-standing MS have ventricular enlargement and/or cortical atrophy.

Many patterns of CT enhancement can be seen, for example ring enhancement, mass formation, oedema, and very complex enhancing lesions. Multifocal enhancing lesions on CT are helpful for demonstrating dissemination in space but are not specific for MS. Any disease that can cause local breakdown in the BBB can produce this pattern, including metastatic neoplasms, cerebral infarctions, brain abscess, primary brain tumours, and other inflammatory neurological diseases.

Magnetic Resonance Imaging in MS

MRI uses a strong magnetic field and radio frequencies in order to produce an image.[10] Hydrogen atoms in the brain will align themselves as dipoles along the magnetic field and

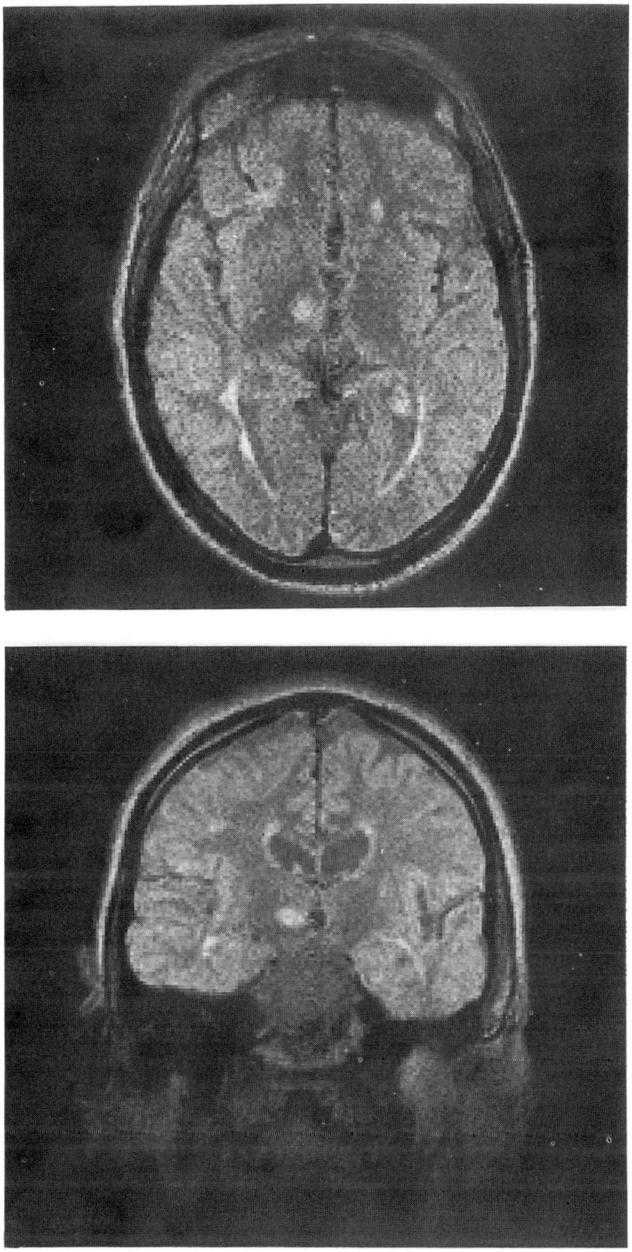

a

b

Fig. 1. *MS lesions in two planes*. There is a lesion in the deep periventricular area of the right hemisphere in two planes (axial, a; coronal, b) (courtesy of Dr. D. Li, UBC MRI Center).

spin like tops, acting as tiny polar magnets. Radio frequencies that are tuned to the resonance frequency of these atoms can cause them to spin at a different angle. The duration of the signal that emanates from the relaxation of that angle can be measured. Computer techniques can then be used to detect not only the location of the source of the signal, but the quantity of atoms in question. Some of the tissue characteristics surrounding the atoms producing the signal are also involved. MRI measures mostly the content of water in the brain, but the molecular state of that water is also reflected in the signal. MRI can also produce images in many planes, allowing lesions to be visualized in more than one dimension. For MS studies the most commonly used image is the spin echo (SE) (Fig. 1). The SE sequence that is most useful is the image in which the lesions of MS stand out as high signal intensity (white) against a darker background. The darker background in the SE image is made up of three contrasting areas: grey matter, white matter, and ventricle. Grey matter is whiter in appearance than normal white matter. The CSF in the ventricles is lower in signal (darker) than normal white matter. This particular combination of signal intensities allows not only for the optimum detection of lesions but also helps to make clear discrimination of lesion from normal white matter and ventricle.

MRI in the diagnosis of MS

The most immediate impact of MRI on MS has been in the area of diagnosis. In 1981 Young *et al.*[11] reported eight patients with clinically definite MS, all of whom had multiple focal areas of abnormality. The sensitivity of MRI for detection of MS lesions was about 10 times greater than that of CT. The high sensitivity was greatest in the brainstem, which is a notoriously poor area for discrimination on the CT scan. MRI cannot distinguish between acute and chronic lesions in MS, but with increasing experience this differentiation may be possible. Enhanced CT scans can easily show BBB disruption. A combination of MRI and HVD CT can identify not only most of the MS lesions (on MRI), but will also distinguish acute lesions by showing focal BBB disruption (on CT). In the future, gadolineum and other paramagnetic contrast materials will also provide a CT-independent MRI marker for BBB disruption.[12]

Typical MS lesions are of high intensity on SE, measure greater than 3 mm in diameter, and are predominantly located in white matter (see Fig. 1). Periventricular and peripheral white matter lesions are characteristic of MS, but only in the proper clinical context.[13] MRI cannot differentiate with certainty between MS lesions, multiple infarcts, and non-specific patterns such as subcortical arteriosclerotic encephalopathy (Binswanger's disease).[14] It is the pattern of lesions that is highly suggestive of MS. However, it must be remembered that tissue characterization by MRI is not yet possible; therefore critical clinical judgement must be used in the interpretation of the scan results.

The MS group at the University of British Columbia has just published a prospective study of the use of MRI in the diagnosis of MS.[15] On the basis of this study there is no doubt that MRI is the most sensitive technique for detecting asymptomatic lesions and demonstrating dissemination in space. Two hundred suspected MS patients were studied, and after one year of follow-up 19 out of those 200 (10%) had converted to clinically definite MS, through having a second clinical episode during the year. Of those 19 patients, 18 were predicted as having MS by MRI scans that were highly suggestive of MS (four or more lesions) during the study. This group of patients is still being followed. Only long-term clinical follow-up will establish the ability of tests such as MRI to predict the diagnosis of clinically definite MS (CDMS) accurately.[16] It was in the clinical categories of optic neuritis and chronic progressive myelopathy (CPM) that MRI and the other clinical tests were most helpful in establishing a diagnosis. About 50 percent of each of those categories could be diagnosed as laboratory supported definite MS by the use of MRI and CSF studies for oligoclonal banding.

MRI assessment of disease activity

Serial MRI scans done in a prospective fashion can provide precise information about the evolution of lesions. We have now studied 23 patients systematically with serial MRI scans, clinical evaluations, and immunological tests.[17-19] There were seven clinical relapses in those 24 patients, each studied for 6 months. In contrast to the rather slow development of clinical relapses (0.6 relapses per patient per year), there were 42 asymptomatic new MRI lesions and 76 significantly enlarging or reappearing MRI lesions, giving a total of 118 active or re-active lesions. Figure 2 shows a series of MRI scans demonstrating the evolution of a new lesion. Patients with chronic progressive disease had twice as many 'active' lesions as did relapsing patients, and they also had more new lesions as well. These serial MRI studies have shown that the frequency of new MRI lesions is 5–10 times the frequency of clinical relapses. Based on this striking MRI phenomenon we propose that, for more accurate assessment of disease activity in future studies, serial MRI scans will be necessary. Even though MRI is unable to identify the actual pathological process in these 'active' and new lesions, the enlarging and resolving lesions must represent a fundamental part of the acute MS process. This technique of serial MRI scanning should decrease the amount of time that must be spent in order to detect significant changes over time. Even though expensive, this method of assessment should increase the objectivity and decrease the amount of time necessary in order to do clinical studies.

The serial studies have shown that disease activity in relapsing MS as detected by MRI is a much more continuously active process than was previously thought. The fact that new lesions are coming and going asymptomatically shows that there is a great deal of disease activity that cannot be detected clinically. The majority of these newly detected lesions diminish in size or actually disappear over time. The usual tempo of evolution of the new lesions is gradual enlargement over 2 to 4 weeks, followed by a gradual decline in size over the next 6 to 10 weeks. In the serial studies there were also 38 instances in which there was MR evidence that some lesions were enlarging while others were decreasing in size simultaneously. These findings suggest that local rather than systemic factors are important in the resolution phase of new lesions.

Quantitation of the extent of the MS process

Early in our experience with MRI in MS we felt that we could use the technique to measure the 'disease burden' in individual patients. We have developed computer-assisted techniques of quantitation that allow the calculation and storage of location, size and intensity of lesions as well as quantitation of the total extent of the disease process.[20] A skilled and experienced technician can outline the MS lesion with a reproducibility error of about 6 percent. The error between different observers can be much greater than that. It is, therefore, important that a single observer be used for any one study in order to minimize systematic quantitation errors. A very critical requirement for serial studies for either quantitative or qualitative assessment of numbers of lesions is the repositioning of the patient. Very careful repositioning is required to minimize artifacts and errors. Errors in repositioning can cause small lesions to fade, appear in adjacent slices, or even to be lost between slices in those machines in which a gap is present between slices.

Our experience has shown that correlation between the extent of disease as measured by MRI and the severity of the disease as determined by clinical scoring methods is poor. Quantitative MRI methods are now being used in clinical trials.[21] We have just completed an alpha lymphoblastoid interferon therapeutic trial in which a quantitative MRI scan was done at entry at 6 months (end of therapy), and at 2 years. Patients were treated with interferon or placebo over 6 months and followed double-blind for 2 years. Analysis of the data at 6 months showed a trend for the extent of the process to be less in the interferon-treated patients.[22] However, the follow-up at 2 years showed that there was no clinical or MRI difference between interferon-treated and placebo-treated patients. Despite the inability to distinguish between groups at 2 years the method was shown to be effective in

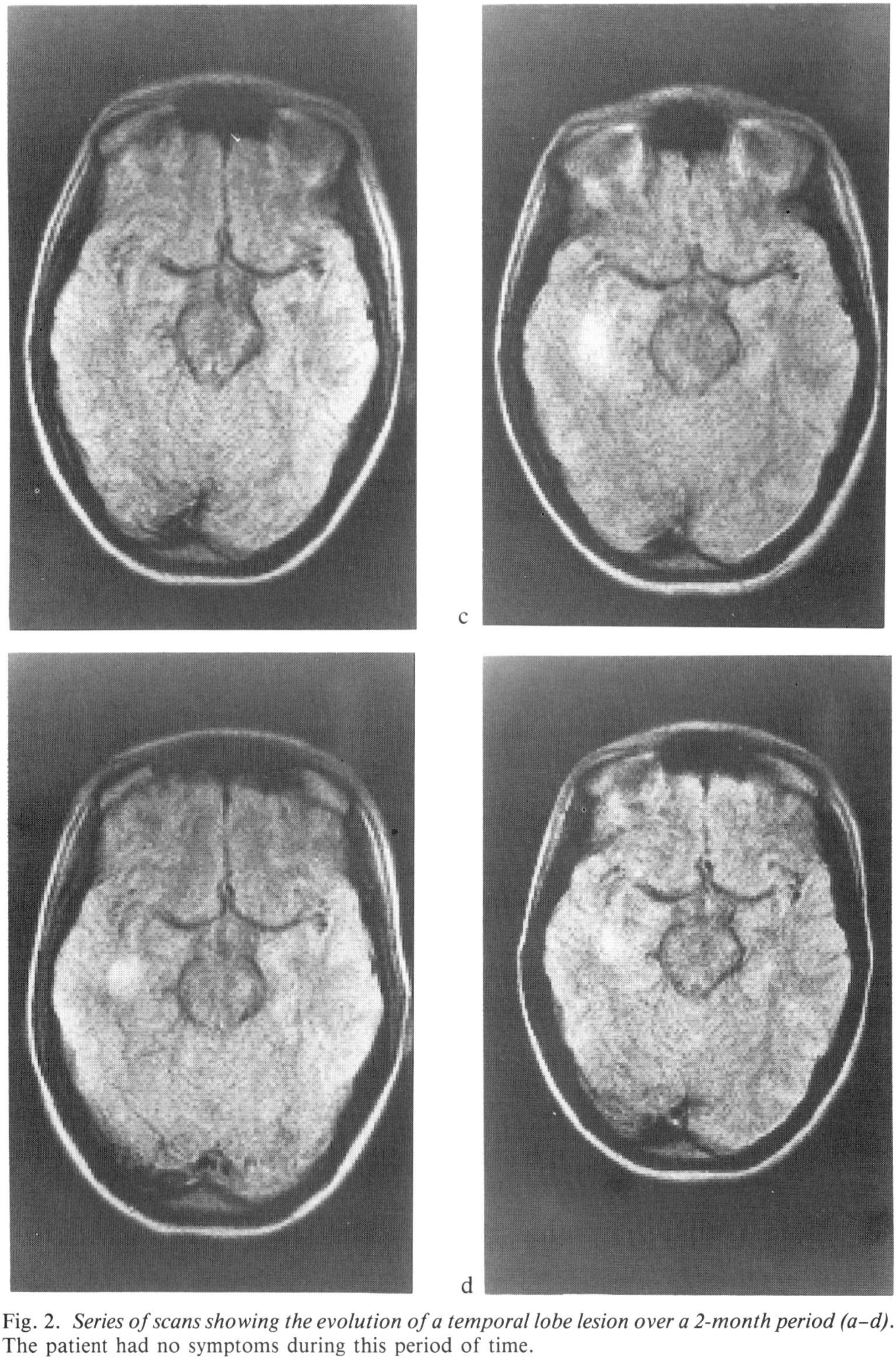

Fig. 2. *Series of scans showing the evolution of a temporal lobe lesion over a 2-month period (a–d).* The patient had no symptoms during this period of time.

measuring changes in extent of disease. The extent of disease in both placebo and interferon-treated patients increased by approximately 20 percent over the 2-year period.

We have also compared the characteristics and extent of lesions in patients with different clinical courses. Koopmans *et al.*[23] compared a group of 32 patients with benign MS with a group of patients with chronic progressive disease, matched for age, sex, and duration of disease. They showed that in 80 percent of these matched pairs there was a heavier 'disease burden' in the progressive patient than in the benign one. However, the total extent of disease overlapped considerably between the two groups and in 20 percent of cases there was a heavier 'disease burden' in the benign patient. This study has supported the long-standing concept that in MS the symptoms cannot be predicted very well from the pathology. The question of clinical expression of MRI lesions and of symptoms without MRI changes was addressed. Instances occurred in which symptoms occurred without lesions and *vice versa*, especially in the brainstem. Since all the new lesions seen on the systematic serial MRI studies have been neurologically asymptomatic it is unclear what features, in addition to location, are necessary to make a lesion symptomatic. Clinical pathological studies in cerebrovascular disease have taught us a great deal about localization as a primary factor in determining 'focal' neurological findings. In MS, there may well be other factors involving the nature of the pathological process that help determine the clinical expression of individual lesions.

The MRI scans in the CP patients showed that there was a striking and characteristic tendency toward periventricular confluence of lesions that was not seen in the scans from benign patients with similar 'disease burden'. Benign MS was much more likely to have lesions scattered throughout the white matter in a 'salt and pepper' appearance.

Pathological findings compared with the MRI appearance

Stewart *et al.*[24] studied eight pathological cases. Lesions as small as 3 mm in diameter could be visualized by MRI. The extent of demyelinated lesions as detected by MRI was very similar to that seen in the pathology. Unfortunately, Stewart's pathological correlation studies have shed little light on the problem of distinguishing acute from chronic lesions. For this reason studies using experimental allergic encephalomyelitis (EAE) have been done. Acute EAE lesions can be seen[25] prior to the onset of clinical signs. There is also a very good correlation between the MRI scan and the actual pathology as to the extent of the EAE. In at least one instance serial studies have shown that MRI lesions can come and go, and then reappear later (all asymptomatic) looking very much like the evanescent new MRI lesions seen in MS patients.[25]

Conclusions

(1) MRI is the most sensitive method of demonstrating dissemination in space for diagnostic purposes. (2) MRI can be used as a quantitative index of the extent of disease. However, the extent of disease as measured by MRI and the location of lesions do not correlate well with clinical severity or symptoms. (3) Frequently performed and carefully repositioned MRI scans can detect a degree of disease activity that is much greater than that suggested by clinical signs and symptoms. (4) In the future, frequent and carefully done quantitative MRI scans are going to be a necessary component of clinical investigations in MS, including clinical trials.

Acknowledgements—Thanks are due to Dr. David Li, Director of our MRI Unit, and to my neurological colleagues at UBC. The studies cited in this paper were supported by the BC Health Care Research Foundation, the MS Society of Canada, and the Jacob W. Cohen Fund for Research in Multiple Sclerosis.

References

1 Stewart, W. A., Hall, L. D., Berry, K., Churg, A., Oger, J., Hashimoto, S. A. & Paty, D. W. (1986): Magnetic resonance imaging (MRI) in multiple sclerosis (MS): Pathological correlation studies in eight cases (abstract). *Neurology* **36**(Suppl 1), 320.

2 Prineas, J. W., Kwon, E. E., Sharer, L. R. & Cho, E-S. (1987): Massive early remyelination in acute multiple sclerosis. *Neurology* **37**(Suppl 1), 109.

3 Poser, C. M., Paty, D. W., Scheinberg, L., McDonald, W. I., Davis, F. A., Ebers, G. C., Johnson, K. P., Sibley, W. A., Silberberg, D. H. & Tourtellotte, W. W. (1983): New diagnostic criteria for multiple sclerosis: Guidelines for research protocols. *Ann. Neurol.* **13**, 227–231.

4 Sears, E. S., McCammon, A., Bigelow, R. & Hayman, L. A. (1982): Maximizing the harvest of contrast enhancing lesions in multiple sclerosis. *Neurology* **32**, 815–820.

5 Fog, T. & Linnemann, F. (1970): The course of multiple sclerosis. *Acta Neurol. Scand.* **46**(Suppl 47), 1-175.

6 Antunes, J. L., Schlesinger, E. B. & Michelsen, W. J. (1974): The abnormal brain scan in demyelinating diseases. *Arch. Neurol.* **30**, 269–271.

7 Brooks, D. J., Leenders, K. L., Head, G., Marshall, J., Legg, N. J. & Jones, T. (1984): Studies on regional cerebral oxygen utilization and cognitive function in multiple sclerosis. *J. Neurol. Neurosurg. Psychiatry* **47**, 1182–1191.

8 Glydensted, C. (1976): Computer tomography of the cerebrum in multiple sclerosis. *Neuroradiology* **12**, 33–42.

9 Ebers, G. C., Vinuela, F. V., Feasby, T. & Bass, B. (1984): Multifocal CT enhancement in MS. *Neurology* **34**, 341–346.

10 Brant-Zawadzki, M. & Norman, D. (1987): *Magnetic resonance imaging of the central nervous system*. New York: Raven Press.

11 Young, I. R., Hall, A. S., Pallis, C. A., Bydder, G. M., Legg, N. J. & Steiner, R. E. (1981): Nuclear magnetic resonance imaging of the brain in multiple sclerosis. *Lancet* **ii**: 1063–1066.

12 Grossman, R. I., Gonzalez-Scarano, F., Atlas, S. W., Galetta, S. & Silberberg, M. D. (1986): Multiple sclerosis: Gadolinium enhancement in MR imaging. *Radiology* **161**, 721–725.

13 Paty, D. W., Asbury, A. K., Herndon, R. M., McFarland, H. F., McDonald, W. I., McIlroy, W. J., Prineas, J. W., Scheinberg, L. C. & Wolinsky, J. S. (1986): Use of magnetic resonance imaging in the diagnosis of multiple sclerosis: Policy statement. *Neurology* **36**, 1575.

14 Zimmerman, R. D., Fleming, C. A., Lee, B. C. P., Saint-Louis, L. A. & Deck, M. D. (1986): Periventricular hyperintensity as seen by magnetic resonance: Prevalence and significance. *AJR* **146**, 443–450.

15 Paty, D. W., Hashimoto, S., Hooge, J., Oger, J., Kastrukoff, L. F., Eisen, A. S., Eisen, K., Purves, S., Brandejs, V., Robertson, W. & Li, D. (1988): Magnetic resonance imaging in the diagnosis of multiple sclerosis (MS): A prospective study of comparison with clinical evaluation, evoked potentials, and oligoclonal banding. *Neurology* **38**, 180–185.

16 Schumaker, G. A., Beebe, G., Kibler, R. F. *et al.* (1965): Problems of experimental trials of therapy in multiple sclerosis: Report by the panel on the evaluation of experimental trials of therapy in multiple sclerosis. *Ann. N.Y. Acad. Sci.* **122**, 522–568.

17 Isaac, C., Li, D., Genton, M., Jardine, C., Grochowski, E., Palmer, M., Kastrukoff, L. F., Oger, J. & Paty, D. W. (1988): Multiple sclerosis: A serial study using MRI in relapsing patients. *Neurology* **38**, 1511–1515.

18 Willoughby, E., Grochowksi, E., Li, D., Oger, J., Kastrukoff, L. & Paty, D. (1989): A second prospective study of MRI in multiple sclerosis. *Ann. Neurol.* **25** 43–49.

19 Koopmans, R., Li, D. K. B., Oger, J. J. F., Kastrukoff, L. F. & Paty, D. W. (1989): Serial MRI studies in chronic progressive MS: An assessment of disease activity. *Ann. Neurol.* (In press).

20 Paty, D. W., Bergstrom, M., Palmer, M., MacFadyen, J. & Li, D. (1985): A quantitative magnetic resonance image of the multiple sclerosis brain (abstract). *Neurology* **35**(Suppl 1), 137.

21 Palmer, M. R., Bergstrom, M., Grochowski, E., Apted, C., Li, D. K., Genton, M., Hashimoto, S. A. & Paty, D. W. (1986): Magnetic resonance imaging (MRI) in multiple sclerosis (MS): Quantitation of changes in the size of lesions over six months in the placebo limb of a therapeutic trial. *Can. J. Neurol. Sci.* **13**, 168.

22 Kastrukoff, L. F., Hashimoto, S. A., Oger, J. J., Sacks, S. L., Li, D. K., Petkau, A., Berkowitz, J. & Paty, D. W. (1987): A trial of Namalwa interferon in the treatment of chronic progressive (CP) multiple sclerosis (MS) 1. Clinical and MRI analysis (abstract). *Can. J. Neurol. Sci.* **14**, 242.
23 Koopmans, R. A., Li, D., Grochowski, E., Cutler, D. & Paty, D. W. (1989): MRI characteristics of benign and chronic progressive multiple sclerosis. *Ann. Neurol.* **25**, 74–81.
24 Stewart, W. A., Hall, L. D., Berry, K. & Paty, D. W. (1984): Correlation between NMR scan and brain slice: Data in multiple sclerosis. *Lancet* **ii**, 412.
25 Stewart, W. A., Alvord, E. C., Hruby, S., Hall, L. D. & Paty, D. W. (1987): Magnetic resonance imaging (MRI) of experimental allergic encephalomyelitis (EAE) in primates. *Am. Assoc. Neuropathol.*, Seattle. Manuscript in preparation.
26 Stewart, W. A.: Personal communication, unpublished results.

7

COGNITIVE IMPAIRMENT IN PATIENTS WITH CLINICALLY ISOLATED LESIONS OF THE TYPE SEEN IN MULTIPLE SCLEROSIS. A PSYCHOMETRIC AND MRI STUDY

M. M. Callanan, S. J. Logsdail, M. A. Ron and E. K. Warrington

The National Hospital for Nervous Diseases, Queen Square, London WC1, UK

Summary

This study reports the performance on psychometric tests of a group of 48 patients with clinically isolated lesions of the type seen in multiple sclerosis (optic neuritis, brain stem and cord lesions). The cognitive functions studied were: 'IQ deficit', verbal and visual memory, abstracting ability, visual and auditory attention and naming ability. The presence of brain pathology was investigated by means of magnetic resonance imaging (MRI). A group of 46 patients with rheumatic and neurological conditions not known to cause brain disease was used for comparison. Normative MRI data were obtained from a group of 40 normal volunteers.

An overall 'Cognitive Ability Index' was significantly worse in patients with clinically isolated lesions when compared with physically disabled controls. IQ deficit and defective auditory attention were the more severely affected variables. These deficits were significantly correlated with the duration of neurological symptoms and with the degree of brain pathology detected by MRI.

Introduction

Cognitive decline in patients suffering from multiple sclerosis (MS) was first mentioned by Charcot over a hundred years ago.[1] Cases of rapidly progressive dementia attributed to the presence of widespread lesions in the white matter have also been reported.[2]

However, the systematic study of the cognitive abnormalities which might be present in a large number of patients with definite MS has only been attempted recently.

Deterioration in non-verbal skills, [3,4] memory,[5–7], and abstracting ability[8] has now been documented in patients with definite MS, sometimes occurring during the early stages of the disease. Attempts have also been made to correlate these deficits with the presence of brain pathology as detected by computerized tomography,[9,10] or with non-specific functional abnormalities, eg decreased blood flow as measured by positron emission tomography.[11]

Magnetic resonance imaging (MRI) has made it possible to detect MS lesions with much greater sensitivity than previous techniques,[12] enabling us to make more accurate clinico-pathological correlations. It has also made possible the study of brain pathology in patients with clinically isolated lesions of the type known to occur in MS, namely optic neuritis, and brain stem and cord lesions. Ormerod *et al.*,[13] using MRI, have found lesions in brain areas other than those responsible for the presenting symptoms in over half of these patients at the time of the initial presentation. Optic neuritis, the best studied of these clinically single lesions, is the first manifestation of MS in about 20 percent of cases and approximately three-quarters of those with this initial presentation go on to develop definite MS.[14] Prospective follow-up studies have not been performed in those with brain stem or cord lesions, but it appears likely that a similar proportion ultimately develop MS.[15]

The cognitive performance of patients with clinically isolated lesions has only been studied in a handful of cases[16] and the possibility that subtle psychometric abnormalities may be one of the earliest counterparts of brain pathology remains to be explored. Clinically isolated lesions provide an unique opportunity to study cognitive abnormalities before the severe physical limitations of the disease become apparent, thus avoiding some of the methodological problems that make interpretations of test results difficult in those with definite MS.[17]

We report here a study of the psychometric performance of a group of patients with clinically isolated lesions in whom the presence of brain pathology in areas other than those responsible for the symptoms was examined using MRI. The test battery used in the study was chosen to assess those abilities known to be impaired in patients with definite MS. In addition, tests of attention, a function likely to be impaired in patients with deep white matter lesions, were also used.

Methods

Subjects

Patients with clinically isolated lesions. Forty-eight right-handed patients (18 men and 30 women) with clinically isolated lesions were included in the study. These are referred to as the index group. Fourteen presented with optic neuritis, 16 with brain stem syndromes and 18 with symptoms from a spinal cord lesion. The patients were part of a large cohort undergoing a study of MRI abnormalities in MS at the National Hospital for Nervous Diseases. Their ages ranged from 20 to 61 years, with a mean of 36.4. The diagnosis of clinically isolated lesion of the type commonly found in MS was made after they had undergone appropriate neurological assessment to exclude other possible aetiologies. Special attention was given to the duration of the neurological symptoms and to whether the patients were in exacerbation at the time of testing. Exacerbation was defined, using the Poser criteria,[18] as a symptom or symptoms of neurological disturbance, with or without objective confirmation, lasting more than 24 hours.

Forty-three patients were physically independent, two required walking aids and three were wheelchair-bound. Seven patients were receiving steroids and 14 were taking benzodiazepines (mainly as night sedation) at the time of the study. Subjects were excluded if they had sustained head injuries with a post-traumatic amnesia of more than 24 hours, or if there was evidence of drug or alcohol abuse. Only those whose first language was English and who had received their primary education in the UK were included in the study.

Seventeen patients were in relapse at the time of testing. Corrected visual acuity was normal in all, except for seven with unilateral optic neuritis who were in relapse. Tests of visual attention were not performed by these seven patients.

Control subjects. Two groups of control subjects were assessed for comparison. A physically disabled control group consisted of 46 patients (18 men and 28 women) suffering from neurological or rheumatic conditions not involving the central nervous system. Twenty-two patients had prolapsed intervertebral discs, seven had peripheral neuropathy, five had muscular dystrophy, two had spinal cord tumours, nine had rheumatoid arthritis and one had plantar fascitis. Their ages ranged from 20 to 68 years, with a mean of 39 years. All had normal (corrected) visual acuity and two were left-handed. Two of them were receiving steroids, 27 were on benzodiazepines (mainly as night sedation), and three were on antidepressants at the time of the study.

Subjects in the physically disabled control group were more disabled than the index patients. Thus, only 27 were physically independent, nine required walking aids and 10 used wheelchairs.

A second control group of 40 normal volunteers (21 men and 19 women) was used to obtain normative MRI data. The subjects in this group were officers in the Salvation Army who volunteered to takc part in the study. Their ages ranged from 19 to 64, mean age 39.9 years. The exclusion criteria used for the clinically isolated lesion group were applied to the control subjects.

Psychometric assessment

The following tests were administered to the index patients and to the physically disabled controls.

(1) National Adult Reading Test (NART) and Schonell Graded Word Reading Test. These tests were administered following the standard procedure of Nelson[19] to provide an estimate of premorbid intelligence, and their combined scores were transformed to IQ equivalents.

(2) Weschler Adult Intelligence Scale (WAIS). A shortened version was used[20] and the following subtests administered: Arithmetic, Similarities, Digit Span, Vocabulary (verbal subtests), Picture Completion, Picture Arrangement, and Block Design (performance tests). The results were prorated to yield measures of Verbal, Performance and Full Scale IQ.

The difference between the estimated premorbid IQ and the full scale WAIS IQ was considered as an index of deterioration, hereafter referred to as IQ deficit.

(3) Recognition Memory for Words.[21] This was administered following the standard procedure. The test consists of 50 stimulus words. Recognition memory was tested by presenting each of the words paired with a distractor, the subject being required to make a forced choice between them. The raw score (number of words correctly recognized) was converted to an age corrected scaled score.

(4) Recognition Memory for Faces.[21] Fifty black and white photographs of unfamiliar male faces were the stimuli and the subject was asked to recognize them when each was

paired with a distractor photograph drawn from a similar pool. The raw score (number of faces correctly recognized) was converted to an age corrected scaled score.

(5) Wisconsin Card Sorting Test. The shortened version of this test was used.[22] It consists of one set of stimulus cards and two sets of 24 response cards, the subject being asked to sort them according to one of three attributes in turn (colour, shape or number). The total number of errors was recorded as a measure of abstracting ability.

(6) Speed of Letter Counting. This test is based on a letter cancellation task described by Willison *et al.*[23] and consists of 90 large letters (19 As, Bs and Cs and 17 Ds and Es) arranged randomly in 12 rows and five columns. The time taken to count the As on the page was recorded as a measure of visual attention.

(7) Auditory attention was tested using an adaptation of a vigilance task provided by Kaplan (personal communication).[24] Five groups of 20 letters each were read at a speed of one letter per second and recorded on tape. Embedded among them was the alphabet in the conventional order. The subject was required to make a sign when he heard the first letter of the alphabet, then when he heard the second, etc, until the letter 'z' had been signalled. Prior to testing the subjects were asked to recite the alphabet to ensure that they were familiar with it and they were given a practice run of 20 letters in which the first five letters of the alphabet were embedded. The test was interrupted if the subjects signalled at the wrong letter (false positive errors) or if the correct one was missed (false negative errors) in which case they were told the next letter they should be listening for. The total number of errors, positive and negative, was recorded as a measure of auditory attention.

(8) Graded Naming Test. This object-naming test of graded difficulty,[25] consisting of 30 black and white line drawings, was administered following standardized procedures. The number of objects correctly named was recorded as a measure of naming skill.

The psychometric assessment lasted approximately one and a half hours. The tests were administered in the following order: naming, reading and memory tests, WAIS, tests of abstracting ability and attention tests. Thus, seven psychometric functions were examined: IQ deficit, Verbal Memory, Abstracting Ability, Visual Attention, Auditory Attention and Naming Ability. A grading system (0 to 3) was devised for each of these functions. Grade 0 was assigned to scores at or above the 50th percentile of the control group, Grade 1 to scores falling within the 25th and 50th percentiles of the control group, Grade 2 to scores within the 5th and 25th percentiles, and Grade 3 to scores equal to worse than the 5th percentile of the control group. These grades were summed to provide an overall Cognitive Ability Index. A similar grading system (0–3) based on the distribution of the Cognitive Ability Index scores in the control group was applied to the overall Cognitive Ability Index scores in the isolated lesion group. Thus, a Cognitive Ability Grade 0 represented the summed grades at or above the 50th percentile of the control group, Grade 1 the summed grades between the 25th and 50th percentiles of the control group, etc. This procedure does not rely on the assumption that the various tests measure independent cognitive functions, and permits the combination of scores from different tests in which the units of measurement are not the same.

Motor assessment

A measure of hand function and a measure of the ability to perform everyday tasks were used in the index patients and the physically disabled controls.

(1) Jebsen Hand Function Test. This test[26] comprises eight standardized timed tasks of hand function. Seven of them (writing, maze tracing, card turning, simulated feeding, putting small objects into a can, picking up large light objects, and picking up large heavy

objects) were performed with each hand in turn. The eighth task, assembling nuts and bolts, required the use of both hands. The final score was the sum of the times taken to accomplish the eight tasks.

(2) Activities of Daily Living. Seven standardized motor tasks related to everyday activities were tested: dressing, walking, climbing stairs, bathing, transferring from bed to chair, tea making and feeding. The scoring system was a modification of that used by Haworth & Hollings.[27] The patient's performance on each of these tasks was graded on a four point scale (0 = no assistance needed, 1 = help from others or mechanical aid required, 2 = help from others and mechanical aid required, 3 = unable to attempt or finish task). The final score was the sum of the partial scores.

Psychiatric assessment

Index patients and the physically disabled controls were assessed psychiatrically. The methodology and results of this assessment have been reported elsewhere.[28] The Clinical Interview Schedule (CIS)[29] was used for this purpose. The total score (range 0–33), which includes ratings of subjective symptoms and objective behaviour, was used in the analysis. Patients who scored 14 or more were considered to be psychiatric 'cases'.

MRI assessment

The imager used in the study was a 0.5 tesla Picker superconducting system used to form proton NMR images. The detailed methodology of the scan assessment has been reported elsewhere.[13] Briefly, the presence and size of lesions were examined in seven periventricular areas (body of the ventricles, frontal, temporal and occipital horns, trigone, and 3rd and 4th ventricles) and in the following areas of the brain parenchyma: internal capsule, basal ganglia, and frontal, parietal, temporal and occipital lobes.

Lesions in each of these areas were scored from 0 to 3 depending on the size of their longest diameter (0 = < 2 mm, 1 = 2 to 5 mm, 2 = 5 to 10 mm, 3 = > 10 mm). A total lesion score was obtained by adding the scores of the various areas examined. A 'periventricular' score was obtained by adding the scores of the periventricular areas, a 'frontal' score by adding the scores of the areas around the frontal horns and those of the frontal lobes, and a 'temporal' score by adding the scores of the areas surrounding the temporal horns to those of the temporal and parietal lobes.

MRI scans were obtained in all index patients and in 40 normal controls. In addition 16 randomly-selected physically disabled controls were also scanned as a probe to detect the presence of unsuspected brain pathology. Due to the limited availability of the MRI scanner it was not possible to scan all the subjects in this group.

In most cases the psychometric, psychiatric and motor assessments were carried out on the same day as the MRI scan, but when this was not possible the interval between the clinical and MRI assessments was never more than two weeks. The subject's informed consent was obtained in all cases.

Statistical analysis

Non-parametric statistics were used. This decision was taken because some of the variables were not normally distributed and others, such as the Cognitive Ability Index, were scored on an ordinal scale. Differences between the groups were tested using the Mann-Whitney U-test and the Kruskall-Wallis one way analysis of variance (ANOVA). The Kendall tau test was used to explore correlations between variables. Two-tailed tests of significance were used throughout. The Statistical Package for Social Scientists (SPSS/PC)[30] was used for the analysis.

Results

Psychometric results in patients and physically disabled controls

Patients with optic neuritis, brain stem lesions and cord lesions performed similarly in all psychometric tests (Table 1) and for this reason they were considered as a single group for the main analysis.

As expected there were no significant differences in age, sex or education between index patients and physically disabled controls. Similarly no significant differences in premorbid IQ or current IQ were observed between patients and controls (mean NART scores 110.4 and 109.2 respectively), both groups performing within the normal range (Table 2).

The Cognitive Ability Index of the index patients was also significantly different from that of the controls (respective means 7.15 and 5.3, $P<0.001$), indicating a worse overall performance on psychometric tests.

The specific differences between the groups were explored by comparing the grades obtained on each function (Table 3). Thus, whilst nearly half of the controls scored within Cognitive Ability Grade 0 (good performance), less than a quarter of the patients did so,

Table 1. *Mean scores in patients with clinically isolated lesions.* Results are means (s.d.).

	Optic neuritis (n = 14)	*Brain stem (n = 16)*	*Spinal cord (n = 18)*	*(Kruskal-Wallis ANOVA) (x^2)*	
Premorbid IQ (NART)	112.5 (5.7)	111.5 (6.3)	109.0 (8.1)	2.51	
Full Scale IQ (WAIS)	110.4 (7.5)	106.2 (11.5)	108.1 (10.2)	0.47	
Verbal memory	12.9 (1.8)	11.8 (2.8)	12.1 (2.6)	0.66	
Visual memory	11.2 (3.2)†	11.6 (2.7)	11.1 (3.0)	0.16	
Abstracting ability	5.4 (3.6)	5.7 (3.9)	8.7 (7.6)	1.20	NS
Visual attention	15.8 (2.8)†	14.3 (4.4)	18.0 (7.2)	2.4	
Auditory attention	1.3 (1.8)	2.3 (1.5)	2.8 (4.2)	4.03	
Naming ability	21.6 (3.7)	21.4 (4.8)	22.6 (3.7)	0.68	

NS = not significant
†$n = 7$

Table 2. *Psychometric function scores in patients with clinically isolated lesions and controls.* Results are means (s.d.).

	Clinically isolated lesion patients (n = 48)		*Controls (n = 46)*	
Premorbid IQ	110.7	(6.9)	109.2	(7.8)
Full scale IS (WAIS)	108.0	(10.1)	109.7	(9.9)
IQ deficit	2.2	(7.4)	−0.7	(8.4)
Verbal memory	12.1	(2.5)	12.5	(2.0)
Visual memory	11.3	(2.9)†	12.0	(3.4)
Abstracting ability	6.7	(5.6)	5.8	(5.2)
Visual attention	16.2	(5.4)†	14.1	(3.4)
Auditory attention	2.2	(2.9)	1.2	(2.1)
Naming ability	21.9	(4.0)	21.7	(3.0)

†$n = 41$

Table 3. *Psychometric function grades in patients with clinically isolated lesions and controls.* Results are percent of subjects in each function grade.

	0 (good)		*1 (fair)*		*2 (poor)*		*3 (deficient)*		*Mann–Whitney*
	patients	*controls*	*patients*	*controls*	*patients*	*controls*	*patients*	*controls*	*test (z)*
IQ deficit	33	54	27	28	29	13	10	4	−2.45*
Verbal memory	54	61	19	20	23	17	4	2	−0.80
Visual memory	40	52	33	28	25	13	2	7	−1.11
Abstracting ability	42	52	29	24	27	22	2	2	−0.93
Visual attention	27	52	38	26	27	17	8	4	−2.33*
Auditory attention	25	48	23	30	44	20	8	2	−30.2[‡]
Naming ability	52	37	23	30	15	20	10	2	−1.08

*$P<0.05$; [‡]$P<0.005$

and the patients were three times as likely as the controls to score within Grade 3 (deficient range) (Figure). In addition, the distribution of patients and controls across the grades was significantly different for IQ deficit, and for visual and auditory attention (Table 3).

Clinical features and psychometric test performance

Duration of illness. The controls had been ill for longer than the index patients (mean duration of illness 9.3 and 2.2 years respectively, $P<0.001$). Within the index group 38 out of the 48 patients had had symptoms for less than a year, and only one had been ill for longer than 4 years. The mean duration of illness was shortest for those with optic neuritis (mean 0.93 years), followed by those with brain stem (2.5 years)

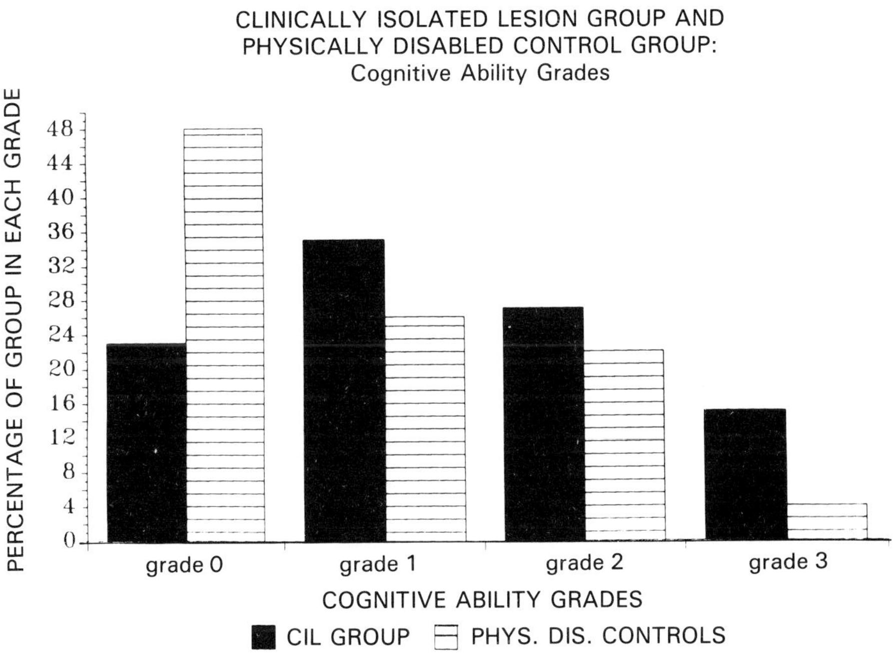

Figure. *Clinically isolated lesion group and physically disabled control group: cognitive ability grades.*

and cord lesions (3 years). These differences between groups reached statistical significance ($P<0.04$).

In the control group the duration of illness was not significantly related to the performance on any of the psychometric tests. In the index group as a whole there was a significant correlation between the duration of neurological symptoms and the performance on visual attention tests ($P<0.05$), and within this group the most significant correlations were found in those with spinal cord lesions who also had the longest duration of symptoms. Thus, the longer the history the greater the impairment in tests of visual attention ($P<0.02$), auditory attention ($P<0.02$), abstracting ability ($P<0.04$), and Cognitive Ability Index ($P<0.05$).

Physical disability. Within the index group, impairment in tests of attention could not be explained as a result of the neurological deficits. Optic neuritis patients with impaired vision were excluded, and those with brain stem syndromes performed the same as the rest of the group in tests of auditory attention (Table 1). Physically disabled controls performed significantly worse than the patients with clinically isolated lesions in Activities of Daily Living ($P<0.05$). Similarly, within the index group those with optic neuritis performed significantly better than the rest on these complex activities ($P<0.005$), even though the group as a whole was only mildly disabled.

There were no differences between the index patients and the physically disabled controls in the test of hand function. Performance on this test was also similar across the three subgroups of patients with clinically isolated lesions. Within the index group significant correlations were found between the speed of hand function and the scores of the psychometric tests with the exception of tests of memory and naming ability. In the physically disabled control group significant correlations, albeit with a different pattern, were also found. Thus, visual memory ($P<0.05$), naming ability ($P<0.05$) and Cognitive Ability Index ($P<0.005$) became worse as hand speed decreased.

Relapses and remissions. The 17 patients who were in relapse at the time of the study had significantly greater IQ deficit than the rest of the group ($P<0.05$). The individual psychometric functions and overall cognitive ability were similar in both groups.

Psychiatric morbidity. Eight out of the 48 index patients were considered to have clinically significant psychiatric symptoms at interview, while this was the case for two out of the 46 physically disabled controls. These differences failed to reach statistical significance, and the same was true for the CIS scores in each group (Mann-Whitney$=0.43$, $P=0.67$).

In the index group there were no significant differences in the psychometric test performance between those who were psychiatrically ill and the rest. In the group as a whole the severity of psychiatric symptoms, as reflected in the CIS score, correlated significantly with the Cognitive Ability Index and visual attention scores, while in the control group similar correlations were obtained with the measure of IQ deficit and the Cognitive Ability Index (Table 4).

Abnormal fatiguability. The subjective experience of fatigue was one of the symptoms rated in the CIS. Patients who scored two or more (range 0–4) were considered to be abnormal. Thirteen out of the 48 index patients and 11 out of the 46 controls were found to have abnormal fatigue ratings. In the index group those with abnormal ratings had significantly worse abstracting ability functions ($P<0.05$) and a worse Cognitive Ability Index

Table 4. *Psychiatric morbidity and psychometric test performance.* Results are correlations with Clinical Interview Schedule score[29] (Kendall tau).

	Patients (n = 48)	*Controls (n = 46)*
IQ deficit	0.05	0.18*
Verbal memory	−0.002	0.00
Visual memory†	−0.008	−0.02
Abstracting ability	0.14	0.08
Visual attention†	0.25*	0.14
Auditory attention	0.09	0.16
Naming ability	0.14	0.15
Cognitive Ability Index	0.20*	0.19*

*$P<0.05$; †$n=41$

($P<0.05$) when compared with the rest of the group, while in the control group greater IQ deficit ($P<0.05$), worse visual attention ($P<0.05$) and Cognitive Ability Index ($P<0.05$) were the main differences.

Psychotropic drugs. There were no significant differences in the performance of psychometric tests between index patients who were receiving psychotropic medication and those who were not. The same was the case for the physically disabled controls.

MRI abnormalities in patients and controls

The MRI abnormalities in patients and controls have been reported elsewhere.[28] Abnormalities were detected in 39 out of the 48 index patients (81%) and in two out of the 16 physically disabled controls. The proportion and type of abnormalities detected in the physically disabled controls were similar to those found in the normal controls, in whom abnormalities were present in five out of 40. In the index patients a periventricular rim of increased signal was the commonest MRI abnormality, often accompanied by discrete lesions in the brain parenchyma. The total lesion score of the group with clinically isolated lesions was significantly different from those of the two control groups (total lesion scores 9.8, 0.71 and 0.52 respectively, $P<0.001$). There were no significant differences in the total lesion scores among the index patient subgroups, but in those with cord lesions the score was significantly correlated to the duration of neurological symptoms ($P=0.02$).

Psychometric tests and MRI abnormalities

Of the individual psychometric functions explored, performance in tests of auditory attention and abstracting ability were significantly correlated with the total lesion score (Table 5). A similar trend was also found for those with more MRI abnormalities to have a poorer overall Cognitive Ability Index, although this correlation failed to reach statistical significance. Furthermore, when those with a Cognitive Ability Grade of 0 (good performance) were compared with those who scored within Grade 3 (deficient performance), the degree of detectable brain pathology was different in the two groups. Thus the total lesion score was three times higher for those in Grade 3 than for those in Grade 0 (mean 21.1 and 6.7, $P<0.05$).

Table 5. *MRI total lesion score and psychometric function scores in patients with clinically isolated lesions.*

	MRI total lesion score (Kendall tau)
IQ deficit	0.11
Verbal memory	−0.02
Visual memory	0.07
Abstracting ability	0.18*
Visual attention	0.01
Auditory attention	0.20*
Naming ability	−0.03
Cognitive ability index	0.16

*$P<0.05$

There were no significant correlations between the results of the psychometric tests and the 'periventricular', 'frontal', and 'temporal' scores.

The two physically disabled controls with MRI abnormalities (aged 51 and 62) were older than the mean age for the group (39 years). One of them suffered from a prolapsed intervertebral disc and the other had a neurofibroma of a spinal root. Their scores on the Cognitive Ability Grade were 1 and 2 respectively.

Discussion

We report here a study of the psychometric deficits encountered in a group of patients with clinically isolated lesions of the type seen in MS in whom the presence of brain pathology has been ascertained by MRI. The results of the study suggest that cognitive impairment can be detected when other manifestations of brain pathology are absent and that attention deficits are the most prominent cognitive abnormalities in these patients. These deficits are related to the duration of the neurological symptoms and are significantly correlated with the overall degree of brain pathology detected using MRI.

The control group used in the study differed from the group with clinically isolated lesions in several important ways and this illustrates the difficulties encountered in trying to match subjects for all the relevant variables. The physically disabled patients had been ill for longer and had greater physical handicaps than those with clinically isolated lesions. However, the speed of hand function, a measure relevant to the performance of psychometric tests, was similar in the two groups. These differences could hardly explain the worse cognitive performance in those with clinically isolated lesions, and if at all relevant they are likely to minimize the differences in test performance between the two groups.

The presence of psychiatric symptomatology is also unlikely to account for the greater cognitive impairment in those with clinically isolated lesions. Psychiatric morbidity was low in both groups and was found to be more closely related to environmental factors than to the presence of brain pathology.[28] The modest correlations found between the severity of psychiatric symptoms and cognitive performance were present in patients and controls, and therefore are unlikely to account for the cognitive differences between the groups.

Abnormal fatiguability, a common complaint in definite MS, is in most cases a primary manifestation of the disease, although in some patients it could be a symptom of depression, systemic illness or a side-effect of drugs. In this study the patients with clinically isolated lesions complained of fatigue as often as the controls. In our study the use of psychotropic medication was the same in both groups and unrelated to test performance. This suggests that fatiguability in the clinically isolated lesion patients, who are less disabled than controls, is partly due to the presence of brain damage. On the other hand, fatigue *per se* is unlikely to account for the differences in cognitive ability between the two groups.

In the only available study of cognitive impairment in patients with clinically isolated lesions, Lyon-Caen *et al.*[16] have described impairment with optic neuritis when compared with a heterogeneous group of patients, some of whom were likely to have been brain-damaged. Their findings are in some way similar to those reported here, although the relationship of cognitive impairment to brain pathology was not explored in that study.

In comparison with patients suffering from definite MS, the cognitive deficits of our patients with clinically isolated lesions are mild. A variety of memory functions, free recall in particular, have been found to be impaired in MS even after a short illness.[6,7] Recognition memory tests were used in our study because they allow the testing of visual and verbal memory using the same technique, something difficult to achieve with tests of free recall, and because they are resistant to the effects of depression.[31] No memory disturbances were found using these tests in our patients, but it would be worthwhile to examine memory functions in greater detail in future studies, as they are likely to be affected early in the course of the disease. The normal performance in tests of naming ability is in keeping with the well preserved language abilities often reported in patients with definite MS. On the other hand, there was a suggestion that a decline in IQ may have been present in our patients, an observation also reported in those with definite MS.[3,32]

Attentional processes have not been explored in patients with definite MS, despite empirical reasons to suspect that they may be impaired in a disease with predominantly subcortical pathology. Moreover, attention is required in the performance of tasks of abstracting ability known to be impaired in definite MS.[3,4,8] In our study measures of auditory and visual attention were impaired in patients with clinically isolated lesions whose performance on a number of other tests was normal, suggesting that this may be one of the most sensitive measures of cognitive impairment in MS.

The cognitive impairment in patients with clinically isolated lesions was best illustrated by the use of the Cognitive Ability Index. By combining the various test scores this overall measure highlights the presence of minor degrees of impairment that would have remained undetected if only single test measures had been used, and removes the need for making multiple comparisons which could have yielded spurious results.

The MRI abnormalities found in this study have been described in detail elsewhere.[28] Briefly, the proportion of MRI abnormalities found in the physically disabled patients was similar to that found in the normal control group and in keeping with previous studies of healthy volunteers ([33] and D. Miller, personal communication, 1987), which have reported the increasing frequency of patchy periventricular high signal lesions with advancing age. The type and distribution of MRI abnormalities in the patients with clinically isolated lesions were similar to those found in definite MS, but the overall amount of detectable pathology was much smaller. In our study the most striking cognitive abnormality, impaired auditory attention, was also the one which correlated most closely with the overall degree of detectable brain pathology, followed by impairment in abstracting ability, a function which is partly dependent on attentional processes. These clinico-pathological correlations were also reflected in the significantly greater degree of brain pathology detected in those with a deficient overall cognitive ability when compared with those with good overall performance. The lack of correlation between the specific functions tested and the indices of focal brain pathology was disappointing. However, these are crude indicators of the extent of MRI abnormalities in large brain regions and it is likely that more accurate delimitation of areas involved in specific cognitive processes and the use of more sensitive magnetization parameters will yield more relevant information.

Finally, the results of the study suggest that in patients with clinically isolated lesions, cognitive impairment is a more reliable indicator of brain pathology than the presence of psychiatric abnormalities[28] or more conventional neurological symptoms or signs. It would also seem possible that in cases of 'silent' or 'benign' MS[34] similar abnormalities might have been elicited if carefully sought.

Acknowledgements—We are indebted to the members of the MRI research group at the National Hospital for Nervous Diseases and to the MS Society for providing the MRI scanner. Ms L. Jones and her colleagues in the Occupational Therapy Department helped with the motor assessment of patients and Dr. T. Shallice gave valuable help with the statistical analysis of the psychometric data. We are also grateful to Professor W. I. McDonald and Professor W. A. Lishman who made helpful comments on the manuscript, and to Mrs T. Guise for typing it. Finally, our thanks are due to all the subjects who took part in the study and their consultants who allowed us to approach them. The study was supported by a grant from the Medical Research Council.

Permission has been received from the Editor of *Brain* and its publishers, Oxford University Press to reprint this article, data from which were accepted for publication in *Brain* in 1988.

References

1 Charcot, J. M. (1977): *Lectures on the diseases of the nervous system*. London: New Sydenham Society.

2 Bergin, J. D. (1957): Rapidly progressive dementia in disseminated sclerosis. *J. Neurol. Neurosurg. Psychiatry* **20**, 285–298.

3 Reitan, R. M., Reed, J. C. & Dyken, M. L. (1971): Cognitive, psychomotor and motor correlates of multiple sclerosis. *J. Nerv. Ment. Dis.* **153**, 218–225.

4 Ivnik, R. J. (1978): Neuropsychological stability in multiple sclerosis. *J. Consult. Clin. Psychol.* **46**, 913–923.

5 Beatty, P. & Gange, J. J. (1977): Neuropsychological aspects of multiple sclerosis. *J. Nerv. Ment. Dis.* **164**, 42–50.

6 Grant, I., McDonald, W. I., Trimble, M. R., Smith, E. & Reed, R. (1984): Deficient learning and memory in early and middle phases of multiple sclerosis. *J. Neurol. Neurosurg. Psychiatry* **47**, 250–255.

7 Rao, S. M., Hammeke, T. A., McQuillen, M. P., Khatri, B. O. & Lloyd, D. (1984): Memory disturbance in chronic progressive multiple sclerosis. *Arch. Neurol.* **41**, 625–631.

8 Parsons, O. A., Stewart, K. D. & Arenberg, D. (1957): Impairment of abstracting ability in multiple sclerosis. *J. Nerv. Ment. Dis.* **125**, 221–225.

9 Rao, S. M., Glatt, S., Hammeke, T. A., McQuillen, M. P., Khatri, B. O., Rhodes, A. M. & Pollard, S. (1985): Chronic progressive multiple sclerosis: relationship between cerebral ventricular size and neuropsychological impairment. *Arch. Neurol.* **42**, 678–682.

10 Rabins, P. V., Brooks, B. R., O'Donnell, P., Pearlson, G. D., Moberg, P., Jubelt, B., Coyle, P., Dalos, N. & Folstein, M. F. (1986): Structural brain correlates of emotional disorder in multiple sclerosis. *Brain* **109**, 585–597.

11 Brooks, D. J., Leenders, K. L., Head, G., Marshall, J., Legg, N. J. & Jones, T. (1984): Studies on regional cerebral oxygen utilisation and cognitive function in multiple sclerosis. *J. Neurol. Neurosurg. Psychiatry* **47**, 1182–1191.

12 Young, I. R., Hall, A. S., Pallis, C. A., Legg, N. J., Bydder, G. M. & Steiner, R. E. (1981): Nuclear magnetic resonance imaging of the brain in multiple sclerosis. *Lancet* **ii**, 1063–1066.

13 Ormerod, I. E. C., Miller, D. H., McDonald, W. I., du Boulay, E. P. G. H., Rudge, P., Kendall, B. E., Moseley, I. F., Johnson, G., Tofts, P. S., Halliday, A. M., Bronstein, A. M., Scaravilli, F., Harding, A. E., Barnes, D. & Zilkha, K. J. (1987): The role of NMR imaging in the assessment of multiple sclerosis and isolated neurological lesions: A quantitative study. *Brain* **110**, 1579–1616.

14 Francis, D. A., Compston, D. A. S., Batchelor, J. R. & McDonald, W. I. (1987): A reassessment of the risk of multiple sclerosis developing in patients with optic neuritis after extended follow-up. *J. Neurol. Neurosurg. Psychiatry* **50**, 758–765.
15 McDonald, W. I. & Silberberg, D. H. (1986): The diagnosis of multiple sclerosis. In *Multiple sclerosis* eds W. I. McDonald & D. H. Silberberg, pp 1–10. London: Butterworth.
16 Lyon-Caen, O., Jouvent, R., Hauser, S., Chaunu, M., Benoit, N., Widlocher, D. & Lhermitte, F. (1986): Cognitive function in recent onset demyelinating diseases. *Arch. Neurol.* **43**, 1138–1141.
17 Rao, S. M. (1986): Neuropsychology of multiple sclerosis: A critical review. *J. Clin. Experimental Neuropsychology* **8**, 503–542.
18 Poser, C. M., Paty, D. W., Scheinberg, L., McDonald, W. I., Davis, S. A., Ebers, G. C., Johnson, K. P., Sibley, W. A., Silberberg, D. H. & Tourtellotte, W. W. (1983): New diagnostic criteria for multiple disseminated sclerosis. *J. Neurol. Neurosurg. Psychiatry* **20**, 285–298.
19 Nelson, H. E. (1982): *Manual for the National Adult Reading Test.* Windsor: NFER–Nelson Publishing Co.
20 Weschler, D. (1955): *Manual for the Wechsler Adult Intelligence Scale.* New York: The Psychological Corporation.
21 Warrington, E. K. (1984): *Recognition Memory Test.* Windsor: NFER–Nelson Publishing Co.
22 Nelson, H. E. (1976): A modified card sorting test sensitive to frontal lobe defects. *Cortex* **12**, 313–324.
23 Willison, J. R., Thomas, D. J., du Boulay, G. H., Marshall, J., Paul, E. A., Pearson, T. C., Ross Russel, R. W., Symon, L. & Wetherley-Mein, G. (1980): Effect of high haematocrit on alertness. *Lancet* **i**, 846–848.
24 Kaplan, E. (1984): Personal communication.
25 McKenna, P. & Warrington, E. K. (1983): *Manual for the Graded Naming Test.* Windsor: NFER-Nelson Publishing Co.
26 Jebsen, R. H., Taylor, N., Treieschmann, R. B., Trotter, M. J. & Howard, L. A. (1969): An objective and standardized test of hand function. *Arch. Phys. Med. Rehabil.* **50**, 311–319.
27 Haworth, R. J. & Hollings, E. M. (1979): Are hospital assessments of daily living activities valid? *Int. Rehabil. Med.* **1**, 59–62.
28 Logsdail, S. J., Callanan, M. M. & Ron, M. A. (1988): Psychiatric morbidity in patients with clinically isolated lesions of the type seen in multiple sclerosis. A clinical and MRI study. *Psychol. Med.* (in press).
29 Goldberg, D. P., Cooper, B., Eastwood, M. R., Kedward, H. B. & Shepherd, M. (1970): A standardized psychiatric interview for use in community surveys. *Br. J. Prev. Soc. Med.* **24**, 18–23.
30 Norusis, M. J. (1986): *SPSS/PC for the IBM PC/XT/AT.* Chicago: SPSS Inc.
31 Coughlan, A. K. & Hallows, S. E. (1984): The use of memory tests in differentiating organic disorders from depression. *Br. J. Psychiatry* **145**, 164–167.
32 Hirschenfang, S. & Benton, J. G. (1966): Note on intellectual changes in multiple sclerosis. *Percept. Mot. Skills* **22**, 786.
33 Gerard, G. & Weisberg, L. A. (1986): MRI periventricular lesions in adults. *Neurology* **36**, 533–536.
34 Gilbert, J. J. & Sadler, M. (1983): Unsuspected multiple sclerosis. *Arch. Neurol.* **40**, 533–536.

8

CORRELATION OF MAGNETIC RESONANCE IMAGING WITH NEUROPSYCHOLOGICAL TESTING IN MULTIPLE SCLEROSIS

Stephen M. Rao,* Gary J. Leo,* Victor M. Haughton,†
Patricia St. Aubin-Faubert* and Linda Bernardin*

*Departments of *Neurology and †Radiology, Medical College of Wisconsin, Milwaukee, WI, USA*

Summary

Previous research has suggested that cerebral lesions observed on magnetic resonance (MR) scans of multiple sclerosis (MS) patients are clinically 'silent'. We examined the validity of this assertion by correlating neuropsychological test performance with the MR imaging findings in 53 MS patients. We used a semi-automated quantitation system to measure three MR variables: total lesion area (TLA), ventricular-brain ratio (VBR), and size of the corpus callosum (SCC). Stepwise multiple regression analyses indicated that TLA was a robust predictor of cognitive dysfunction, particularly for measures of recent memory, abstract/conceptual reasoning, language, and visuospatial problem solving. SCC predicted test performance on measures of mental processing speed and rapid problem solving, while VBR did not independently predict cognitive test findings. These findings suggest that cerebral lesions in MS produce cognitive dysfunction and that MR imaging may be a useful predictor of cognitive dysfunction.

Introduction

Magnetic resonance imaging (MRI) is extremely sensitive for the detection of focal areas of demyelination in patients with multiple sclerosis (MS).[1,2] The clinical significance of these lesions remains unclear. Their correlation with neurological symptoms and degree of disability has been uniformly disappointing,[3-6] prompting the view that MS lesions occur in brain regions that are clinically 'silent'. Others[7,8] have recommended the use of neuropsychological testing to evaluate the possible relationship between cerebral demyelination and cognitive dysfunction.

Two studies[9,10] attempted to relate cognitive dysfunction to lesions identified by MRI. Franklin *et al.*[9] examined 60 patients with chronic progressive MS, and found a significant correlation ($r = 0.35$) between an overall brain lesion score and a summary score derived from a brief cognitive screening battery. Huber *et al.*[10] administered a brief battery of neuropsychological tests to 30 MS patients, nine of whom were classified as 'demented', 11 as having moderate cognitive impairment, and 12 as minimally impaired. These investigators observed no significant group differences on three MR indices: total lesion score, cerebral atrophy, and severity of periventricular involvement. On the fourth index, atrophy of the corpus callosum, the 'demented' patients had significantly higher ratings than the moderate and minimal cognitive impairment groups.

These two studies found significant correlations between MR variables and cognitive testing, yet the strength of the correlations was modest. Three methodological factors may have contributed to their limited success in obtaining meaningful correlations. First, both studies relied on rating scales to measure the size of lesions from MR scans. Rating scales by definition are subjective and prone to human error. In addition, rating scales provide a more restricted range of data values than quantitative systems that measure lesions in area units; this restricted range may seriously limit the size of obtained correlations. Second, both studies used brief cognitive screening examinations. MS does not produce a uniform decline of all cognitive skills;[7,11] although these brief batteries covered a number of cognitive functions, they may have missed salient cognitive deficits. A more comprehensive neuropsychological examination may be more successful in measuring those cognitive functions that are influenced by MS-related cerebral pathology. Finally, cognitive test performance is affected by education and age.[12] Thus relatively uneducated or older patients may be classified as impaired on testing when they are functioning close to their premorbid level. Conversely, highly educated or younger patients may have experienced declines in cognitive performance that were undetected because their performance remained in the 'average' range. Neither study attempted to control for these potential confounds either experimentally or statistically.

In the present study we administered a comprehensive neuropsychological test battery to a representative sample of MS patients from the community. Size of cerebral lesions and the degree of ventricular and corpus callosum atrophy were quantified from MR scans. Clinicopathological relationships were evaluated using multivariate statistical procedures which adjust for premorbid differences in cognitive ability.

Methods

Patients

We randomly recruited MS patients from a membership listing of a local MS society. A review of medical records allowed determination of the basis for the diagnosis of MS. We excluded patients not meeting the criteria of Poser *et al.*[13] for definite or probable MS and patients with a history of alcohol/drug abuse or nervous system disorder other than MS. Once enrolled, a neurological examination verified the Poser diagnostic classification and rated patients with regard to disease course, length of symptoms, severity of global dementia (Mini-Mental State examination),[14] and physical disability (Kurtzke Expanded Disability Status Scale; EDSS).[15] Patients subsequently underwent neuropsychological testing and MR scanning over a two-day period to minimize fatigue. Patients gave informed consent according to institutional guidelines.

MR imaging

Imaging was performed on a commercial 1.5 Tesla superconductive magnet (General Electric Signa System). We obtained sagittal images with a repetition time (TR) of 600 msec, an echo time (TE) of 20 msec, and a 5 mm slice thickness. These images enabled the selection of a series of axial slices with a TR of 2 sec and TEs of 25 and 80 msecs. The technical factors included two excitations, a 128 × 256 matrix, a 5 mm slice thickness, and a 1 mm 'skip' between slices.

One investigator, without knowledge of the clinical and neuropsychological profiles of the patients, obtained measurements of total lesion area (TLA), size of the corpus callosum (SCC), and ventricular-brain ratio (VBR). This was accomplished by tracing the outlines of lesions and cerebral structures on the MR scanner computer console. Software routines available on the G. E. Signa System computed the area (in cm^2) subtended by each tracing. We recorded sizes of the following cerebral structures: the third and lateral ventricles from

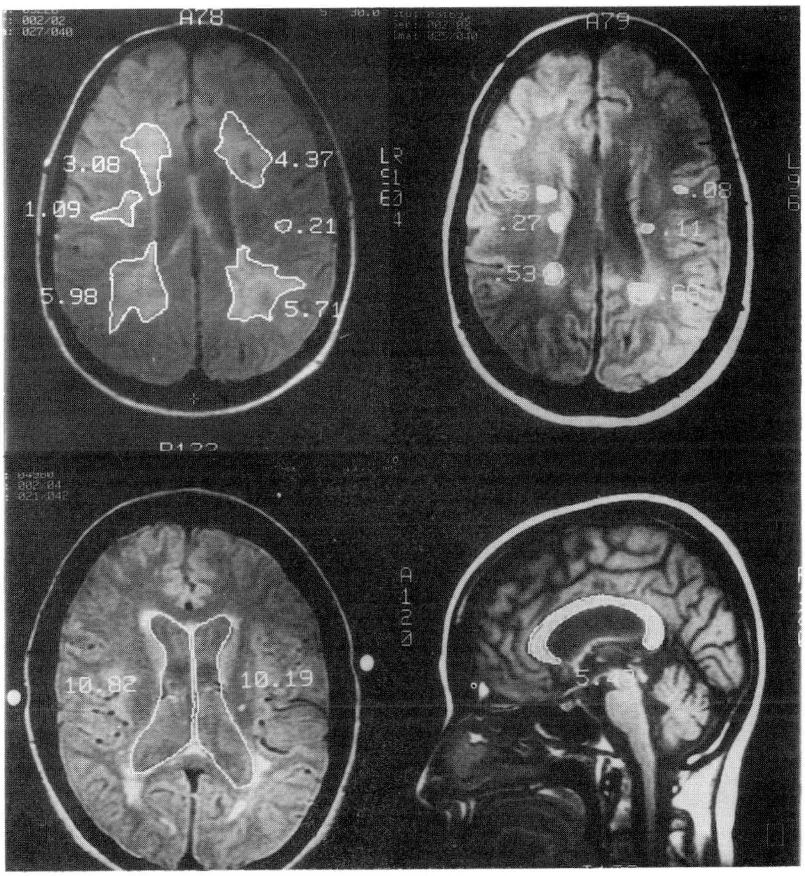

Fig. 1. *Measurement of lesions.* The two top scans illustrate the outlining and measurement of lesions (in cm^2) for two patients. Note that while the number of lesions (6) is the same for both patients, major differences exist in the total lesion area (20.4 *vs* 2.0 cm^2) and average lesion size (3.4 *vs* 0.3 cm^2). The lower left scan demonstrates the outlining and measurement of the lateral ventricular spaces (used to compute ventricular-brain ratios), while the lower right scan shows the measurement of the corpus callosum from the midsagittal scan.

axial slices, the entire area of the brain for each axial slice in which the third and/or lateral ventricles could be visualized, and the corpus callosum from the midsagittal slice (see Fig. 1). We computed TLA by adding all measurements of lesion size for a given patient and VBR by dividing the sum of the ventricular measurements by the sum of the brain area measurements.

Neuropsychological tests

The neuropsychological test battery consisted of measures of verbal intelligence, memory, abstract/conceptual reasoning, attention/concentration, language, and visuospatial skills. We specifically chose tests that do not require fine visual acuity or motor speed/dexterity.

Verbal intelligence was assessed with the six subtests constituting the Verbal subscale of the Wechsler Adult Intelligence Scale-Revised (WAIS-R)[16]: Vocabulary, Information, Digit Span (see attention/concentration tests below), Comprehension, Similarities, and Arithmetic.

The recent memory tests consisted of the Buschke Verbal Selective Reminding Test,[17] the 7/24 Spatial Recall Test,[18,19] and the Story Recall Test.[20] The Story Recall Test was administered with immediate, 1-hour, and 24-hour delayed recall. We assessed remote memory by asking the subjects to recall the past eight U. S. presidents (President's Test).[20] The Brown-Peterson Interference Test[21,22] assesses the rate of forgetting from immediate memory; the stimuli were three 3-letter words, the delay intervals were 0, 3, 9, and 18 sec, and the interference task consisted of counting backwards by threes during the delay interval. We computed rate of forgetting by subtracting the number of words correctly recalled after an 18 sec delay (max = 15) from words recalled after no delay (max = 15).

Tests of abstract/conceptual reasoning skills consisted of the Wisconsin Card Sorting Test,[23] Booklet Category Test,[24] Standard Raven Progressive Matrices,[25] and Stroop Colour/Word Interference Test[26] (total time to read a colour list was subtracted from total time to read the colour-word list).

Assessment of attention/concentration skills included forward and backward digit span (WAIS-R instructions), simple *versus* two-choice complex reaction time (RT)[27] (simple RT was subtracted from complex RT), Sternberg Memory Scanning Task[28] (which yields two measures: slope, a measure of mental processing speed; and y-intercept, a measure of overall motor reaction time), and Paced Auditory Serial Addition Test[29] (using two conditions based on different rates of stimulus presentation; for the 'easy' condition, 60 single digits were presented at 3 sec intervals, and for the 'hard' condition, 60 digits were presented at 2 sec intervals).

The language measures used in this study primarily assessed expressive abilities. These included: an abbreviated (15-item) version of the Boston Naming Test,[20] Controlled Oral Word Association Test (F-A-S version), [30] and Category Word Generation Test (animal names version).[20]

We assessed visuospatial skills with the Hooper Visual Organization Test[31] and three Benton *et al.*[32] tests: Judgment of Line Orientation, Facial Recognition, and Visual Form Discrimination.

Data analysis

Statistical analyses were performed with the microcomputer version of the Statistical Package for the Social Sciences.[33] We performed separate stepwise multiple regression analyses for each of the 34 cognitive measures, which served as the dependent (criterion) variables. The independent (predictor) variables were age, education, TLA, VBR, and SCC. Age and education were always entered on the first step to adjust for their effects on the cognitive variables and to adjust for the effects of age on VBR (see below).

We employed cluster analysis (nearest centroid sorting method)[34] to classify patients into two subgroups: patients with relatively substantial cognitive impairment ('Impaired') *versus* those with relatively minimal impairment ('Intact'). Thus we selected a two group cluster solution *a priori*, with the analysis performed on the 10 cognitive test variables shown to be the most sensitive to cognitive dysfunction in MS patients from previous neuropsychological investigations.[19,35-39] The variables included: long-term storage: Selective Reminding Test; immediate recall: Story Recall Test; number of perseverative errors: Wisconsin Card Sorting Test; total errors: Booklet Category Test; number correct: Raven Progressive Matrices; time difference between colour/word and word reading: Stroop Interference Test; T-score: Hooper Visual Organization Test; scanning rate: Sternberg Memory Scanning Task; percent correct: hard form of the Paced Auditory Serial Addition Test; and total words generated: Controlled Oral Word Association Test. As in earlier studies,[19] we performed cluster analysis on the standardized residual scores generated from regression analyses relating cognitive test scores (criterion variable) with demographic (predictor) variables (ie age, education, sex, and occupation). This method minimizes individual differences in premorbid ability levels.

Results

A total of 59 patients were enrolled in the study. We eliminated six patients from the final analysis: four did not complete MR scanning due to claustrophobia, one did not meet the Poser criteria after completion of the neurological examination, and one had a brainstem arteriovenous malformation diagnosed by MRI. All but two patients were in clinical remission at the time of evaluation. Table 1 presents demographic and illness characteristics for the patient sample.

MR measurements

We obtained TLA and VBR measurements for all 53 patients and SCC measurements for 45 of 53 patients in whom precise midline saggital cuts were available. All but one patient

Table 1. *Clinical characteristics of MS sample (n = 53).*

Sex (males/females)	13/40	
Age, years (mean)	43.9	(range 27–61)
Education, years (mean)	13.6	(range 8–20)
Occupation (6-pt scale, mean)	4.1	(range 2–6)
Estimated premorbid IQ[a] (mean)	106.1	(range 89–118)
Length of symptoms, years (mean)	12.2	(range 1–33)
Years since diagnosis (mean)	7.8	(range 1–28)
Kurtzke Expanded DSS (mean)	3.8	(range 0–8)
Diagnostic Category (nos):		
Clinically definite	37	(70%)
Laboratory definite	10	(19%)
Clinically probable	6	(11%)
Clinical Course (nos):		
Relapsing-remitting	21	(40%)
Chronic-progressive	10	(19%)
Chronic-stable	21	(39%)
Benign	1	(2%)
Mini-Mental State (max = 30) (mean)	28.8	(range 12–30)

[a] Estimated from demographic variables using regression formula derived from WAIS-R standardization sample.[40]

Table 2. *Results of stepwise multiple regression analyses, showing MR variables (in rank order) making significant contributions to the prediction of cognitive test performance after partialling out age and education.* No MR variable significantly predicted results of (Memory) President's Test, Brown–Peterson Interference Test; (Attention/Concentration) Digit span, Reaction Time.

Cognitive test	*MR Variable*	*Partial*	R^2	*Change* R^2
(1) Verbal intelligence				
WAIS-R Verbal IQ	SCC	0.37	0.39	0.10*
Vocabulary	TLA	−0.31	0.41	0.06*
Comprehension	SCC	0.38	0.23	0.13*
Arithmetic	SCC	0.39	0.31	0.13†
(2) Memory				
Selective Reminding Test:				
Long term storage	TLA	−0.40	0.31	0.13†
Consistent long term retrieval	TLA	−0.38	0.32	0.12*
7/24 Spatial Recall Test:				
Total recall	TLA	−0.31	0.9	0.07*
Delayed recall	TLA	−0.35	0.22	0.11*
Story Recall Test:				
Immediate recall	TLA	−0.41	0.37	0.13†
1 hour delayed recall	TLA	−0.43	0.37	0.14†
24 hour delayed recall	TLA	−0.48	0.43	0.17†
(3) Abstract/conceptual reasoning				
Wisconsin Card Sorting Test:				
Categories completed	TLA	−0.49	0.41	0.19‡
Perseverative errors	TLA	0.44	0.34	0.16†
Booklet Category Test:				
Total errors	SCC	−0.48	0.41	0.18†
	TLA	0.34	0.48	0.07*
Raven Progressive Matrices:				
Number correct	TLA	−0.54	0.55	0.18†
Stroop Interference Test:				
Colour/word–word condition (sec)	TLA	0.38	0.18	0.14*
(4) Attention/concentration				
Sternberg Memory Scanning Task:				
Scan rate (msec per digit)	SCC	−0.48	0.33	0.20†
Y intercept (msec)	- - -			
Paced Auditory Serial Addition Test:				
Percent correct—easy	- - -			
Percent correct—hard	SCC	0.40	0.32	0.13†
(5) Language				
Abbreviated Boston Naming Test:				
Total correct	TLA	−0.35	0.16	0.12*
Controlled Oral Word Association Test:				
Total words generated	SCC	0.39	0.24	0.14*
Category Word Generation:				
Total words generated	TLA	−0.38	0.23	0.13*

Table 2. (continued)

Cognitive test	*MR Variable*	*Partial*	R^2	*Change* R^2
(6) Visuospatial skills				
Hooper Visual Organization Test:				
T-score	TLA	0.49	0.25	0.24‡
Judgment of Line Orientation Test:				
Number correct	SCC	0.47	0.30	0.20†
Facial Recognition Test:				
Number correct	TLA	−0.34	0.24	0.10*
Visual Form Discrimination Test:				
Number correct	TLA	−0.35	0.22	0.11*

MR = magnetic resonance; Partial = partial correlations between cognitive and MR variables correcting for age, education, and previously entered MR variables; R^2 = multiple R squared; Change R^2 = improvement in R^2 achieved by adding MR variable(s) to prediction equation; SCC = size of corpus callosum; TLA = total lesion area; - - - = no MR variable significantly predicted cognitive variable.
* $P<0.05$; † $P<0.01$; ‡ $P<0.001$.

had at least a single cerebral lesion. The following summarizes the mean (s.d.) and range of values for the three MR variables: TLA 21.7 (23.9) cm^2, 0–95; VBR 0.044 (0.027), 0.006–0.133; and SCC 4.49 (1.28) cm^2, 1.01–7.08. These three variables correlated significantly with each other: r = 0.61 for TLA *vs* VBR ($P<0.001$); r = −0.46 for TLA *vs* SCC ($P<0.01$); and r = −0.48 for VBR *vs* SCC ($P<0.001$). Age correlated significantly with VBR (r = 0.42, $P<0.01$), but not with TLA or SCC.

Stepwise regression analysis

Table 2 presents the results of stepwise multiple regression analyses for each of the cognitive variables. This table includes only those MR variables making a significant ($P<0.05$) contribution to the prediction of cognitive test performance. The partial correlation coefficients (labelled 'Partial' in Table 2) represent the magnitude of the relationship between the cognitive and MR variables after the effects of age and education are statistically removed. The sign of the coefficient indicates whether the relationship was positive or negative. The partial correlations ranged from −0.31 (Vocabulary subtest of the WAIS-R with TLA) to −0.54 (Raven Progressive Matrices and TLA).

The cumulative amount of shared variance between the dependent and independent variables was estimated by the squared multiple correlation coefficient (R^2 in Table 2). Multiplying this value by 100 gives the percent of variance in each cognitive measure accounted for by the MR variable(s), age, and education. The amount of shared variance ranged from 55 percent (a strong relationship) for the Raven Progressive Matrices to 16 percent (a weak relationship) for the Abbreviated Boston Naming Test.

The amount of shared variance accounted for by the specific addition of the MR variable to the regression equation, excluding the effects of age and education, was estimated by the change in the squared multiple correlation coefficient (Change R^2 in Table 2). These values ranged from 24 percent ($P<0.001$) for the Hooper Visual Organization Test to 6 percent ($P<0.05$) for the Vocabulary subtest.

At least one MR variable significantly ($P<0.05$) predicted 25 of 34 (74%) cognitive test variables. Of these 25 cognitive variables, TLA predicted 18 and SCC predicted eight; two MR variables, SCC and TLA, predicted performance on the Booklet Category Test, an abstract/conceptual reasoning test. VBR did not *independently* predict any of the cognitive variables.

TLA was the best predictor of performance on measures of recent memory and abstract/conceptual reasoning, while SCC was the best predictor of information processing speed (scan rate on the Sternberg test), sustained attention and rapid problem solving (hard form of the Paced Auditory Serial Addition Test), and mental arithmetic (Arithmetic subtest of the WAIS-R). Various tests of verbal intelligence, linguistic processes and visuospatial problem solving skills were predicted by both TLA and SCC (see Table 2).

Cluster analysis

Table 3 presents the results of the two group cluster solution. Nineteen patients (36%) performed below expectations on neuropsychological testing ('Impaired' group; mean cluster centre = −0.691), while 34 patients (64%) performed at or slightly above expectations ('Intact' group; mean cluster centre = +0.358). No significant group differences were observed on demographic variables and on estimated *premorbid* Verbal IQ derived from demographic variables.[40]

In contrast, we observed a significant group difference on *current* WAIS-R Verbal IQ ($t = 4.13$, d.f. = 51, $P < 0.0001$). There was also a small but statistically significant difference between the clusters on the Mini-Mental State ($t = 2.55$, d.f. = 51, $P < 0.02$); mean values for both groups were in the non-demented range, however.[14] While the two groups did

Table 3. Results of cluster analysis.

Variable	*Intact (n = 34)*	*Impaired (n = 19)*
Sex (males/females)	10/24	3/16
Age, years: mean (s.d.)	43.7 (7.7)	44.2 (10.0)
Education, years	13.9 (2.3)	13.0 (2.4)
Occupation (6 pt scale)	4.3 (1.3)	3.8 (1.7)
Estimated Premorbid Verbal IQ[a]	107.8 (5.8)	104.7 (8.4)
Tested verbal IQ	105.6 (11.6)	91.8 (11.6)‡
Mini-Mental State	29.5 (0.9)	27.6 (4.2)*
Currently employed: number (percent)	15 (44%)	3 (16%)*
Length of symptoms, years	12.0 (7.8)	12.6 (7.1)
Years since diagnosis	7.6 (7.1)	8.1 (5.8)
Kurtzke Expanded DSS	3.4 (2.2)	4.6 (1.9)
Diagnosis Category (nos):		
Clinically definite	25	12
Laboratory definite	5	5
Clinically probable	4	2
Clinical Course (nos):		
Relapsing-remitting	16	5
Chronic-progressive	6	4
Chronic-stable	11	10
Benign	1	0
MR Variables:		
TLA	12.2 (13.4)	38.6 (29.2)‡
VBR	0.037 (0.020)	0.057 (0.033)†
SCC[b]	4.9 (1.0)	3.6 (1.3)†

TLA = total lesion area; VBR = ventricular-brain ratio; SCC = size of corpus callosum.
*$P < 0.05$; †$P < 0.01$; ‡$P < 0.001$.
[a] Estimated from demographic variables using regression formula derived from WAIS-R standardization sample.[40]; [b]
[b] Intact: $n = 30$; impaired: $n = 15$.

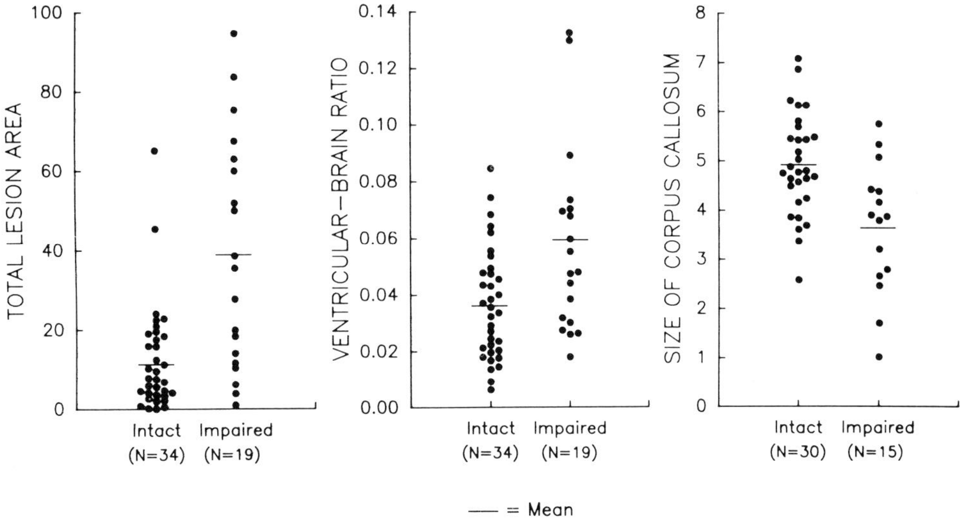

Fig. 2. *Total lesion area, ventricular-brain ratio, and size of the corpus callosum for cognitively intact and impaired MS patients.*

not differ in duration of symptoms, disease course, or overall physical disability (Kurtzke EDSS), it is noteworthy that patients in the cognitively impaired group were less likely to be employed than patients in the cognitively intact group (16% *versus* 44%, respectively; $\chi^2 = 4.36$, d.f. = 1, $P < 0.04$).

Also listed in Table 3 are the means and standard deviations of the three MR variables for the two clusters. The impaired group had significantly greater TLA ($P < 0.001$) and VBR ($P < 0.01$), and smaller SCC ($P < 0.01$), than the intact group. Figure 2 presents MR values for individual subjects in each cluster. Of the three MR variables, the TLA variable achieved the greatest degree of cluster separation. Ten of 12 patients with TLA greater than 30 cm^2 were members of the cognitively impaired cluster; conversely, 32 of 41 patients with TLA less than 30 cm^2 were in the cognitively intact group.

Discussion

The results of this study demonstrate a strong relationship between the severity of cerebral pathology on MR scan and cognitive dysfunction in MS patients. The robust MR correlations in the present study contrast with the weak or non-existent correlations obtained in previous studies that have relied on the neurological examination as the indicator of cerebral involvement.[3-6] This may be explained by the neurological examination underestimating cognitive dysfunction in MS patients when compared to results derived from neuropsychological testing.[38]

We observed the strongest clinicopathological correlations on measures of recent memory and abstract/conceptual reasoning, skills that are most often impaired in MS patients.[7,11] We also observed significant correlations between MR variables and skills infrequently studied in MS patients: rapid and sustained problem solving, language, and visuospatial skills. These findings suggest that cerebral demyelination may be associated with a wider range of cognitive dysfunction than previously suspected.

The relationship between the degree of corpus callosum atrophy and performance on tasks requiring sustained attention and rapid problem solving raises the possibility that such performance depends on precisely timed inter-hemispheric communication that is disrupted by demyelinated callosal fibre tracts. This observation also suggests that specific cognitive processes may be disrupted by demyelinating lesions involving relatively focal structures.

Ventricular size did not independently predict cognitive performance beyond what could be predicted by measures of lesion area and callosal atrophy. In a previous study,[41] we demonstrated statistically significant, albeit weak, correlations between ventricular enlargement and cognitive performance in MS patients. Ventricular enlargement presumably results from 'thinning' of the periventricular white matter as a consequence of demyelination. As such, ventricular enlargement is an indirect, and presumably late, marker of disease activity within the cerebrum.

Results of the cluster analysis suggest that if the total lesion load on MR scan is excessive (arbitrarily defined as greater than 30 cm^2 in the present study), there is a high probability that an MS patient will have cognitive impairment. The practical significance of identifying cognitive dysfunction is highlighted by the observation that MS patients with cognitive impairment are less likely to be employed than patients without cognitive impairment. We observed this relationship despite the fact that the two clusters did not differ in severity of physical disability, duration of illness, or disease course.

We found no relationship between duration of illness and degree of MR abnormalities; furthermore, this study, as well as others, [19,42,43] found no relationship between duration of illness and severity of cognitive disturbance. These negative findings may result from limitations of the cross-sectional research design used in this and other studies. Longitudinal studies are therefore needed to examine the natural history of cognitive dysfunction in MS, particularly in light of disease progression as visualized by MRI.

Acknowledgements—Reprinted with permission from an article first published in *Neurology*. Supported in part by a Research Career Development Award (KO4 NS1055) and a Research Grant (RO1 NS22128) from NINCDS to Dr Rao. The assistance of the Multiple Sclerosis Society of Milwaukee is gratefully appreciated.

References

1 Lukes, S. A., Crooks, L. E., Aminoff, M. J. *et al.* (1983): Nuclear magnetic resonance imaging in multiple sclerosis. *Ann. Neurol.* **13**, 592–601.

2 Young, I. R., Hall, A. S., Pallis, C. A., Legg, N. J., Bydder, G. M. & Steiner, R. E. (1981): Nuclear magnetic resonance imaging of the brain in multiple sclerosis. *Lancet* **ii**, 1063–1066.

3 Jacobs, L., Kinkel, W. R., Polachini, I. & Kinkel, R. P. (1986): Correlations of nuclear magnetic resonance imaging, computerized tomography, and clinical profiles in multiple sclerosis. *Neurology* **36**, 27–34.

4 Kirshner, H. S., Tsai, S. I., Runge, V. M. & Price, A. C. (1985): Magnetic resonance imaging and other techniques in the diagnosis of multiple sclerosis. *Arch. Neurol.* **42**, 859–863.

5 Reese, L., Carr, T. J., Nicholson, R. L. & Lepp, E. K. (1986): Magnetic resonance imaging for detecting lesions of multiple sclerosis: Comparison with computed tomography and clinical assessment. *Can. Med. Assoc. J.* **135**, 639–643.

6 Edwards, M. K., Farlow, M. R. & Stevens, J. C. (1986): Multiple sclerosis: MRI and clinical correlation. *A.J.N.R.* **7**, 595–598.

7 Rao, S. M. (1986): Neuropsychology of multiple sclerosis: A critical review. *J. Clin. Exp. Neuropsychol.* **8**, 503–542.

8 van den Burg, W., van Zomeren, A. H., Minderhoud, J. M., Prange, A. J. A. & Meijer, N. S. A. (1987): Cognitive impairment in patients with multiple sclerosis and mild physical disability. *Arch. Neurol.* **44**, 494–501.

9 Franklin, G. M., Heaton, R. K., Nelson, L. M., Filley, C. M. & Seibert, C. (1988): Correlation of neuropsychological and magnetic resonance imaging findings in chronic/progressive multiple sclerosis. *Neurology* **38**, in press.
10 Huber, S. J., Paulson, G. W., Shuttleworth, E. C. *et al.* (1987): Magnetic resonance imaging correlates of dementia in multiple sclerosis. *Arch. Neurol.* **44**, 732–736.
11 Peyser, J. M. & Poser, C. M. (1986): Neuropsychological correlates of multiple sclerosis. In *Handbook of clinical neuropsychology, vol. 2*, eds S. B. Filskov & T. J. Boll, pp 364–397. New York: Wiley.
12 Prigatano, G. P. & Parsons, O. A. (1976): Relationship of age and education to Halstead Test performance in different patient populations. *J. Consult. Clin. Psychol.* **44**, 527–533.
13 Poser, C. M., Paty, D. W., Scheinberg, L. *et al.* (1983): New diagnostic criteria for multiple sclerosis: Guidelines for research protocols. *Ann. Neurol.* **13**, 227–231.
14 Folstein, M. F., Folstein, S. E. & McHugh, P. R. (1975): Mini-Mental State: A practical method for grading the cognitive state of patients for the clinician. *J. Psychiatr. Res.* **12**, 189–198.
15 Kurtzke, J. F. (1983): Rating neurologic impairment in multiple sclerosis: An expanded disability status scale (EDSS). *Neurology* **33**, 1444–1452.
16 Wechsler, D. (1981): *Manual for the Wechsler Adult Intelligence Scale-Revised.* New York: Psychological Corporation.
17 Buschke, H. & Fuld, P. A. (1974); Evaluating storage, retention, and retrieval in disordered memory and learning. *Neurology* **24**, 1019–1025.
18 Barbizet, J. & Cany, E. (1968): Clinical and psychometrical study of a patient with memory disturbances. *Int. J. Neurol.* **7**, 44–54.
19 Rao, S. M., Hammeke, T. A., McQuillen, M. P., Khatri, B. O. & Lloyd, D. (1984); Memory disturbance in chronic progressive multiple sclerosis. *Arch. Neurol.* **41**, 625–631.
20 Caine, E. D., Bamford, K. A., Schiffer, R. B., Shoulson, I. & Levy, S. (1986): A controlled neuropsychological comparison of Huntington's disease and multiple sclerosis. *Arch. Neurol.* **43**, 249–254.
21 Brown, J. (1958): Some tests of the decay theory of immediate memory. *Q. J. Exp. Psychol.* **10**, 12–21.
22 Peterson, L. R. & Peterson, M. J. (1959): Short-term retention of individual verbal items. *J. Exp. Psychol.* **58**, 193–198.
23 Heaton, R. K. (1981): *Wisconsin Card Sorting Test manual.* Odessa, FL: Psychological Assessment Resources.
24 DeFilippis, N. A. & McCampbell, E. (1979): *The Booklet Category Test manual.* Odessa, FL: Psychological Assessment Resources.
25 Raven, J. C. (1960): *Guide to the standard progressive matrices.* London: H. K. Lewis.
26 Stroop, J. R. (1935): Studies of interference in serial verbal reactions. *J. Exp. Psychol.* **18**, 643–662.
27 Benton, A. L. (1977): Interactive effects of age and brain disease on reaction time. *Arch. Neurol.* **34**, 369–370.
28 Sternberg, S. (1969): Memory scanning: Mental processes revealed by reaction-time experiments. *Am. Scientist* **57**, 421–457.
29 Gronwall, D. M. A. (1977): Paced auditory serial-addition task: A measure of recovery from concussion. *Percept. Mot. Skills* **44**, 367–373.
30 Benton, A. L. & Hamsher, K. deS. (1976): *Multilingual aphasia examination.* Iowa City: University of Iowa.
31 Hooper, H. E. (1958): *The Hooper Visual Organization Test manual.* Los Angeles: Western Psychological Services.
32 Benton, A. L., Hamsher, K. deS., Varney, N. R. & Spreen, O. (1983): *Contributions to neuropsychological assessment: A clinical manual.* New York: Oxford University Press.
33 Norusis, M. J. (1986): *SPSS/PC+ for the IBM PC/XT/AT.* Chicago: SPSS, Inc.
34 Anderberg, M. R. (1973): *Cluster analysis for applications.* New York: Academic Press.
35 Rao, S. M., Hammeke, T. A. & Speech, T. J. (1987): Wisconsin Card Sorting Test performance in relapsing-remitting and chronic-progressive multiple sclerosis. *J. Consult. Clin. Psychol.* **55**, 263–265.
36 Rao, S. M., Leo, G. J. & St. Aubin-Faubert, P. (1988): On the nature of memory disturbance in multiple sclerosis. *J. Clin. Exp. Neuropsychol.* **10**, 48.

37 Rao, S. M., St. Aubin-Faubert, P. & Leo, G. J. (1989): Information processing speed in patients with multiple sclerosis. *J. Clin. Exp. Neuropsychol.* **11**, in press.
38 Peyser, J. M., Edwards, K. R., Poser, C. M. & Filskov, S. B. (1980): Cognitive function in patients with multiple sclerosis. *Arch. Neurol.* **37**, 577–579.
39 Lincoln, N. B. (1981): Discrepancies between capabilities and performance of activities of daily living in multiple sclerosis patients. *Int. Rehabil. Med.* **3**, 84–88.
40 Barona, A., Reynolds, C. R. & Chastain, R. (1984): A demographically based index of premorbid intelligence for the WAIS—R. *J. Consult. Clin. Psychol.* **52**, 885–887.
41 Rao, S. M., Glatt, S., Hammeke, T. A. *et al.* (1985): Chronic progressive multiple sclerosis: Relationship between cerebral ventricular size and neuropsychological impairment. *Arch. Neurol.* **42**, 678–682.
42 Marsh, G. (1980): Disability and intellectual function in multiple sclerosis. *J. Nerv. Ment. Dis.* **168**, 758–762.
43 Ivnik, R. J. (1978): Neuropsychological test performance as a function of the duration of MS-related symptomatology. *J. Clin. Psychiatr.* **39**, 304–307.

9

CEREBRAL BLOOD FLOW AND COGNITIVE FUNCTIONING IN MULTIPLE SCLEROSIS

Henry Nielsen†, Lone Knudsen*, Egon Stenager*, Niels Kjaer Olsen†, Erna Enevoldsen† and Knud Jensen*

*From the Department of †Neurology and * the Neuropsychiatric Research Unit, Odense University Hospital, Odense, Denmark*

Summary

Seventeen patients with multiple sclerosis (MS) and 17 matched controls underwent neuropsychological testing. Another control group and 16 of the MS patients had cerebral blood flow measurement with the ^{133}xenon inhalation technique.

The mean scores for the group of MS patients and their matched controls were very similar on six of seven subtests from the WAIS-R, but the MS patients performed significantly worse than the controls on tests of verbal learning and memory, visual recognition memory, visuo-motor speed, and mental agility. There was no significant difference in mean flow values for the group of MS patients and the second control group.

In the group of MS patients higher resting cerebral blood flow was generally associated with better test performance, and test results on the whole correlated better with indices of posterior flow than with indices of anterior flow.

The results from this study, together with evidence from the literature, suggest that blood flow decrement, when found, is secondary to cerebral dysfunction caused by the disease. Presumedly, blood flow changes do not occur until intellectual impairment has become general.

Introduction

It is well documented that cognitive deficits can be associated with multiple sclerosis (MS), even in patients with MS of less than two years' duration.[1–4] Memory is one of the most consistently impaired cognitive functions in patients with MS,[5] but impaired 'abstract reasoning', reduced problem solving ability due to perseverative tendencies,[6] poor 'verbal fluency', and slowing of cognitive processing time also occur in a substantial number of MS patients.

It has been shown that intellectual impairment of various aetiologies is associated with reduced regional cerebral blood flow (CBF). This applies to Alzheimer's disease and multi-infarct dementia,[7,8] intracranial bypass candidates,[9] individuals exposed to organic solvents,[10] abstinent alcoholics,[11] and also to persons with other diseases characterized by degenerative cerebral changes.[12]

Only a few studies of CBF in patients with MS are available. Scheinberg *et al.*[13] found that mean values for cerebral blood flow did not differ from the corresponding values for a group of normal controls. In a more recent study Yamaguchi *et al.*[14] used the ^{133}xenon inhalation method and found the F_1 values (the fast clearing compartment) to be reduced in a group of six demented MS patients compared with age-matched normal volunteers or with non-demented patients with MS. Swank *et al.*[15] also employed the ^{133}xenon inhalation method in a study of 71 patients aged 20 to 71 years. In patients in the age range 25–40 years the CBF was equal to or even higher than in normal controls. The CBF of patients of advancing age then decreased rapidly, whereas it remained essentially unchanged in age-matched normal controls. In an even more recent study, CBF was determined in 15 MS patients 'in remission'.[16] Their mean age was 44 years and the flow was measured by means of positron emission tomography. Blood flow was significantly reduced in MS patients compared to a group of normal controls, and the mean IQ was 3.38 points lower than the estimated premorbid mean IQ. The patients scored in the impaired range, especially on a 'forced-choice faces test' and on a verbal fluency test, but no attempt was made to correlate neuropsychological test results and flow indices.

The present study was aimed at determining the CBF and neuropsychological functioning in a group of MS patients. By application of a considerably more comprehensive test battery than in the previous studies, and by using the 32-detector ^{133}xenon inhalation technique, an attempt was made to measure cognitive functioning, cerebral blood flow and, if present, the interrelationship between test performance and flow.

Patients and methods

From a group of 47 patients who were living independently in their own homes and who fulfilled the diagnostic criteria for definite MS proposed by Poser *et al.*[17] seventeen (10 females, 7 males) volunteered to participate in CBF assessment. This subgroup underwent clinical neurological evaluation, and all patients were found to be in a stable condition. Two were employed under sheltered conditions, the rest of the patients were unemployed. The mean age was 40.0 years (36–45 years) and the mean score on the Kurtzke Disability Status Scale was 4.17 (3–6). The self-reported duration of the illness was 12.6 years (4–27 years), and the mean number of years since the establishment of an unequivocal diagnosis was 6.7 years. In five cases the disease had a relapsing-remitting course; in nine cases the course was progressive but had previously been characterized by exacerbations and remissions; two patients were in a chronic stable phase and in only one patient was there a chronic, progressive course.

The study comprised two control groups. Each MS patient was matched with a cerebrally intact individual of the same sex, and of about the same age and socioeconomic status. The mean age for this control group was 39.6 years (35–45 years). From the hospital staff another control group was assembled, totalling 16 subjects with a mean age of 37.4 years (30–43 years). This group consisted of nine females and seven males. The MS patients and their matched controls underwent a neuropsychological test battery which consisted of the following tests: seven subtests from the WAIS-R,[18] Auditory Verbal Learning Test (five learning trials and free recall after 15 minutes),[19] Story Recall,[20] Recurring Figures Test,[21] Visual Gestalt Test,[22] Symbol Digit Modalities Test (SDMT),[23] and Trail Making Test A and B.[24]

The MS patients and the subjects from the second control group had their CBF measured by means of the ^{133}xenon 32-detector inhalation technique. The mean initial slope index (ISI)[25] was calculated from five frontal and seven posterior detectors both for the left and the right hemisphere—excluding four central detectors. CBF measurements were corrected to a PCO_2 of 37 mm Hg, close to the mean PCO_2 value for both groups combined. In most cases this correction caused only small changes in the flow values.

Flow results from one of the MS group (a female patient) were discarded because of technical defects, and in another MS case the left frontal flow was calculated from only four detectors (one detector 'dropped out').

Results

Table 1 shows that the mean scores for the group of MS patients and their matched controls were very similar on six of the seven subtests from the WAIS-R. On the subtest 'similarities' the MS patients scored significantly higher ($P<0.01$, paired t-test) than the control group. However, the mean score on this test for a group of 76 normal individuals (normative neuropsychological data for our own clinical use were provided from this sample) with a mean age of 34.9 years was 18.48 (s.d. 4.59), and consequently the control group in this study had an untypically low mean score, while the MS patients analogously scored higher than 'expected'. From this it follows that the significant difference between means was most likely due to chance.

On all the neuropsychological tests except for the visual gestalt test the MS patients performed significantly worse than the control group. In particular, the patients' scores were not as good as those of the control group on the Recurring Figures Test, a visual memory

Table 1. *Tests of cognitive function in patients with multiple sclerosis (MS) and controls.* Results are means (s.d.).

	MS	*Control*	*t (df = 16)*
Information	19.82 (4.67)	19.41 (4.57)	0.381
Digit Span	11.00 (4.29)	11.94 (2.61)	−0.813
Vocabulary	50.65 (12.78)	51.59 (7.72)	−0.355
Arithmetic	11.65 (4.62)	12.41 (4.54)	−0.796
Similarities	20.53 (4.11)	16.29 (5.08)	2.949‡
Picture Arrangement	10.65 (5.88)	12.71 (5.12)	−1.120
Block Design	27.47 (9.86)	29.71 (10.08)	−0.617
AVLT, total	42.47 (10.08)	49.24 (5.44)	−2.368*
AVLT, delayed	8.88 (2.70)	10.94 (2.36)	−2.728†
Story, immediate	8.82 (2.51)	11.03 (2.94)	−2.871†
Recurring Figures	30.00 (7.12)	40.53 (8.55)	−3.889‡
Visual Gestalt			
Immediate	3.88 (3.92)	2.35 (1.97)	T = 42.5[a]
Learning	5.47 (7.68)	2.71 (2.93)	T = 42[a]
Retention	5.41 (4.56)	5.47 (4.81)	T = 59.5[a]
SDMT	32.38 (11.62)	48.31 (11.80)	−4.461§
Trail Making A	62.69 (24.40)	33.06 (12.49)	3.997‡
Trail Making B	130.56 (71.17)	76.94 (25.64)	2.714†

AVLT: Auditory Verbal Learning Test. SDMT: Symbol Digit Modalities Test.
*$P<0.05$, †$P<0.02$, ‡$P<0.01$, §$P<0.001$
[a]Wilcoxon's matched-pairs signed-ranks test

Table 2. *Scores in the five learning trials of the Auditory Verbal Learning Test.* Results are means (s.d.).

	MS	*Control*
1	5.12 (1.54)	6.18 (1.38)
2	7.24 (2.08)	9.24 (1.35)
3	9.24 (2.41)	10.47 (1.37)
4	9.88 (2.64)	11.29 (1.45)
5	11.00 (2.67)	12.06 (1.71)

Table 3. *Initial slope index (ISI) values in the four cerebral quadrants in MS and control groups.* Results are means (s.d.).

	MS	*Control*	*t*
Right frontal	49.413 (7.03)	49.275 (9.27)	−0.047
Left frontal	48.688 (5.98)	48.750 (8.42)	0.024
Right posterior	46.205 (5.96)	46.652 (7.77)	0.182
Left posterior	46.304 (6.02)	46.777 (7.77)	0.193

test ($P<0.01$), and on measures of visuo-motor speed, mental agility, and visual scanning ability (SDMT: $P<0.001$; Trail Making A: $P<0.01$; Trail Making B: $P<0.02$).

In Table 2 the mean scores from the five learning trials on the Auditory Verbal Learning Test are presented. The MS patients' learning rate was similar to that of the control group, but they consistently learned less than the controls.

Table 4. *Correlations between cognitive test results and cerebral flow measurements.*

	Right frontal	*Left frontal*	*Right posterior*	*Left posterior*
Information	0.076	0.072	0.206	0.169
Digit Span	−0.180	−0.170	0.024	−0.040
Vocabulary	0.292	0.293	0.429	0.396
Arithmetic	0.121	0.116	0.231	0.203
Similarities	0.182	0.199	0.323	0.311
Picture Arrangement	0.193	0.233	0.266	0.270
Block Design	0.093	0.128	0.272	0.248
AVLT, total	0.471	0.455	0.529*	0.493
AVLT, delayed	0.274	0.455	0.342	0.339
Story, immediate	0.427	0.452	0.577†	0.529*
Recurring Figures	0.164	0.207	0.257	0.270
Visual Gestalt				
Immediate	−0.567*	−0.590†	−0.685‡	−0.677‡
Learning	−0.468	−0.487	−0.574*	−0.560*
Retention	−0.109	−0.176	−0.250	−0.257
SDMT	0.222	0.215	0.336	0.342
Trail Making A	−0.045	−0.051	−0.209	−0.200
Trail Making B	−0.306	−0.316	−0.454	−0.434

AVLT = Auditory Verbal Learning Test; SDMT = Symbol Digit Modalities Test
*$P<0.05$, †$P<0.02$, ‡$P<0.01$

Table 3 details the mean ISI values from the four cerebral quadrants. A multivariate test (application of Hotelling's T^2 statistic) indicated a non-significant group difference ($F_{4,27} = 0.268$), and differences between corresponding mean flow values were also non-significant as determined by subsequent t-tests.

In Table 4 the correlations between test results and flow indices are presented. With the exception of three of the four correlation coefficients between flow values and the digit span test all correlations were in the 'expected' direction, ie the higher the flow the better the performance. The correlations between flow indices and scores on three of the four memory tests (AVLT, Story Recall, and Visual Gestalt Test) were significant, and it is obvious that correlations between test scores and posterior flow values were generally higher numerically than the correlations between test scores and anterior flow values.

Discussion

The performance of a group of MS outpatients with only moderate physical impairment was not as good as that of a group of age- and sex-matched normal controls on a series of neuropsychological tests. However, their general premorbid intellectual capacity was essentially preserved. Specifically, the neuropsychological investigation uncovered reduced verbal learning ability (primarily reduced acquisition rate), impaired logical memory and visual recognition memory, and slowing of cognitive and visuomotor speed.

Cerebral blood flow was found to be very similar to the flow values in cerebrally intact individuals of the same age and sex, which is in agreement with the results from a recent study comprising 71 MS patients.[15] Sixty-eight of these 71 patients were reportedly neuropsychologically unimpaired.

Scheinberg *et al.*[13] also found no difference in CBF measurements between a group of 20 MS patients with a mean age of 42 years (mean duration of illness 11.3 years) and a group of normal controls, but they found evidence of 'organic brain damage' in the 12 patients who were evaluated psychologically. However, these patients were only tested with the Rorschach test, and the diagnosis of 'brain damage' may have been doubtful.

Reduced CBF in MS patients has, however, been demonstrated in other studies. Yamaguchi *et al.*[14] measured the CBF in six patients with obvious dementia and a mean age of 39 years (duration of illness was not indicated) and found the flow reduced compared with age-matched normal volunteers. Similarly, Brooks *et al.*[16] determined CBF in a group of 15 MS patients with a mean age of 44 years (mean duration of illness 11.8 years) and found it reduced compared to a group of normal controls. Neuropsychological impairment as well as reduced general intelligence was also shown in a majority of the patients. The subjects included in these two latter studies were obviously more severely impaired intellectually than the 17 patients in the present study, or the patients who had CBF measured by Swank *et al.*[15]

Hence the available evidence suggests that reduced CBF in a majority of MS patients cannot be demonstrated until 10 to 15 years after the emergence of the first symptoms[15] and not until the cognitive decline has developed into general intellectual impairment.

In the group of MS patients with normal CBF, higher flows were generally associated with better test performance. Correlations were highest with results from the neuropsychological tests which are considered to be among the most sensitive measures of brain function (learning and memory tests, trail making B). Generally the correlations between posterior flow values and test results were higher than between anterior flow values and test results.

In this study we were unable to determine whether there existed a closer relationship between CBF values and brain functioning in the group of MS patients than in individuals with unimpaired intellectual capacity.

Acknowledgements—This work was supported by Fonden for Scleroseramte på Fyn and the Danish Multiple Sclerosis Society. We wish to thank Jesper Boldsen, PhD, for assisting with the statistical analyses.

References

1 Lyon-Caen, O., Jouvent, R., Hauser, S., Chaunu, M.-P., Benoit, N., Widlöcher, D. & Lhermitte, F. (1986): Cognitive function in recent-onset demyelinating diseases. *Arch. Neurol.* **43**, 1138–1141.

2 Peyser, J. M. & Poser, D. M. (1986): Neuropsychological correlates of multiple sclerosis. In *Handbook of clinical neuropsychology*, vol. 2, eds S. B. Filskov & T. J. Boll, pp 364–397. New York: John Wiley.

3 Ron, M. A. (1986): Multiple sclerosis: psychiatric and psychometric abnormalities. *J. Psychosom. Res.* **30**, 3–11.

4 van den Burg, W., van Zomeren, A. H., Minderhoud, J. M., Prange, A. J. A. & Meijer, N. S. A. (1987): Cognitive impairment in patients with multiple sclerosis and mild physical disability. *Arch. Neurol.* **44**, 494–501.

5 Rao, S. M. (1986): Neuropsychology of multiple sclerosis: a critical review. *J. Clin. Exp. Neuropsychol.* **8**, 503–542.

6 Rao, S. M., Hammeke, T. A. & Speech, T. J. (1987): Wisconsin card sorting test performance in relapsing-remitting and chronic-progressive multiple sclerosis. *J. Consult. Clin. Psychol.* **55**, 263–265.

7 Barclay, L., Zemcov, A., Blass, J. P. & McDowell, F. (1984): Rates of decrease of cerebral blood flow in progressive dementias. *Neurology* **34**, 1555–1560.

8 Rogers, R. L., Meyer, J. S., Mortel, K. F., Mahurin, R. K. & Judd, B. W. (1986): Decreased cerebral blood flow precedes multi-infarct dementia, but follows senile dementia of Alzheimer type. *Neurology* **36**, 1–6.

9 Brown, G. G., Ewing, J. R., Weiss, S. M., Robertson, W. M. & Welch, K. M. A. (1983): Neuropsychological correlates of regional cerebral blood flow in candidates for extracranial to intracranial bypass. *J. Cereb. Blood Flow Metab.* **3**, S594–S595.

10 Arlien-Søborg, P., Henriksen, L., Gade, A., Gyldensted, C. & Paulson, O. B. (1982): Cerebral blood flow in chronic toxic encephalopathy in house painters exposed to organic solvents. *Acta Neurol. Scand.* **66**, 34–41.

11 Berglund, M., Hagstadius, S., Risberg, J., Johanson, T. M., Bliding, Å. & Mubrin, Z. (1987): Normalization of regional cerebral blood flow in alcoholics during the first 7 weeks of abstinence. *Acta Neurol. Scand.* **75**, 202–208.

12 Risberg, J. (1980): Regional cerebral blood flow measurements by ^{133}Xe-inhalation: methodology and applications in neuropsychology and psychiatry. *Brain Lang.* **9**, 9–34.

13 Scheinberg, P., Blackburn, L. I., Kaim, S. C. & Stenger, C. A. (1953): Cerebral circulation and metabolism in multiple sclerosis. *Arch. Neurol. Psychiatry* **70**, 260–267.

14 Yamaguchi, F., Meyer, J. S., Yamamoto, M., Sakai, F. & Shaw, T. (1980): Noninvasive regional cerebral blood flow measurements in dementia. *Arch. Neurol.* **37**, 410–418.

15 Swank, R. L., Roth, J. G. & Woody, D. C. (1983): Cerebral blood flow and red cell delivery in normal subjects and in multiple sclerosis. *Neurol. Res.* **5**, 37–59.

16 Brooks, D. J., Leenders, K. L., Head, G., Marshall, J., Legg, N. J. & Jones, T. (1984): Studies on regional cerebral oxygen utilisation and cognitive function in multiple sclerosis. *J. Neurol. Neurosurg. Psychiatry* **47**, 1182–1191.

17 Poser, C. M., Paty, D. W., Scheinberg, L., McDonald, W. I., Davis, F. A., Ebers, G. C., Johnson, K. P., Sibley, W. A., Silberberg, D. H. & Tourtellotte, W. W. (1983): New diagnostic criteria for multiple sclerosis: guidelines for research protocols. *Ann. Neurol.* **13**, 227–231.

18 Wechsler, D. (1981): *WAIS-R manual.* New York: Harcourt Brace Jovanovich.

19 Lezak, M. D. (1983): *Neuropsychological assessment*, 2nd edn. New York: Oxford University Press.

20 Barbizet, J. & Cany, E. (1969): A psychometric study of various memory deficits associated with cerebral lesions. In *The pathology of memory*, eds G. A. Talland, N. C. Waugh, pp 49–64. New York: Academic Press.

21 Kimura, D. (1963): Right temporal lobe damage. *Arch. Neurol.* **8**, 264–271.

22 Anderson, R. (1976): Verbal and visuo-spatial memory. *Scand. J. Psychol.* **17**, 198–204.
23 Smith, A. (1978): *Symbol digit modalities test*. Los Angeles: Western Psychological Services.
24 Reitan, R. M. (undated): *Trail making test*. Manual for administration and scoring.
25 Risberg, J., Ali, A., Wilson, E. M., Wills, E. L. & Halsey, J. H. (1975): Regional cerebral blood flow by ^{133}Xenon inhalation. *Stroke* **6**, 142–148.

IV

COGNITION AND NEURO-OPHTHALMOLOGICAL FINDINGS

10

THE IMPACT OF 'PRIMARY' VISUAL EFFECTS ON NEUROPSYCHOLOGICAL PERFORMANCE IN MULTIPLE SCLEROSIS

Lone Knudsen, P. Elbøl, Egon Stenager, Knud Jensen and K. Work

Clinical Neuropsychiatric Research Unit, Departments of Clinical Psychology, Neurology, Psychiatry and Ophthalmology, Odense University Hospital, Odense, Denmark

Summary

Specific ophthalmological defects seen in a sample of 20 MS patients were compared with results of neuropsychological assessment in order to evaluate their influence on test performance. The neuropsychological status of the 20 MS patients was compared with 20 controls, matched for age, social status and level of education.

Subgroups presenting pathological findings were identified on optic disc appearances, colour vision and visual fields. Patients presenting pathological findings on one or more of these dimensions performed less well on tests requiring vision than patients in whom ophthalmological findings were normal.

The relatively poor performance in patients with ophthalmic defects is likely to be due to disturbed visual perception.

Introduction

A number of studies on MS have indicated that the visual system is vulnerable to demyelination.[1–3] Loss of colour vision, paleness of the optic disc, disturbance in eye movement and defects in the visual field have been found in relation to MS[4–7] and other clinical and subclinical deficits have occasionally been observed.[8–11] Reduced visual evoked potentials (VEP) have frequently been reported and sub-clinical disturbances of information processing speed have been suggested.[12–14]

Neuropsychological examination has shown decline in non-verbal memory tests and in other material requiring vision, for example, reproduction of visual patterns in drawings by MS patients lacked detail and were of low quality.[15] In MS it seems to be an open question whether patients with primary visual defects perform more poorly in neuropsychological tests that require vision. We have therefore carried out analyses of test performance of 20 MS patients to clarify the impact of primary visual deficits on neuropsychological results.

Methods

The 20 MS patients were selected from a sample of patients with definite multiple sclerosis from among whom patients with severe nystagmus and tremor of the head and upper limbs were excluded. From a pool of healthy persons a group of 20 controls was selected and matched for age, sex and social status.

Ophthalmological assessment of the MS patients was carried out on reading vision, normal distance vision, colour vision, Hess Lee Screen, and computer-assisted static perimetry using the Octopus 2000 perimeter, which determines local visual thresholds by an adaptive strategy. The MS group and the control group were given a neuropsychological test programme tabulated in the sequence of results. Analysis of the variance within the MS group and the control group on neuropsychological test performance using t-test or rank sum test was carried out. For the ophthalmological variables the MS group was divided into two subgroups, one with normal findings and one of pathological findings. All the psychological test results registered were analysed, in order to describe the possible impact of pale discs, loss of colour vision, visual field defects and abnormal eye movements on the neuropsychological results.

In the assessment of visual fields, the score of fluctuation or ability to cooperate was registered. Within the MS group no significant correlations were found between self-reported traits of depression on Beck Depression Inventory or self-reported traits of anxiety on the STAI-trait Inventory and the estimates of ability to cooperate in the visual field examination.

A possible impact of abnormal eye movements on neuropsychological results was analysed, but no significant deviation was found, although 11 patients had pathological findings on the Hess Lee Screen.

Co-variant analyses were carried out on scores of all the ophthalmological variables and on neuropsychological memory test results. No significant explanatory values were found on verbal memory tests.

Results and discussion

In the MS group there were 15 women and 5 men. Mean age (range) was 38.7 (25–45) years, disability scale score 3.3 (1–6), duration of illness 11.7 (4–26) years, and time since diagnosis 6.5 (1–14) years. In Table 1 the MS and control groups are compared for performance on the WAIS-R subtests. There was no significant difference between the mean

Table 1. *WAIS-R subtests (raw score).* Results are means (s.d.).

	MS patients (n = 20)	*Controls (n = 20)*
Information	18.40 (5.24)	20.20 (3.78)
Digit Span	11.30 (3.84)	12.15 (2.39)
Vocabulary	48.35 (13.40)	52.85 (7.44)
Arithmetic	11.30 (4.10)	13.40 (4.06)
Similarities	19.35 (5.23)	17.10 (4.02)
Picture Arrangement	11.00 (6.09)	13.15 (4.49)
Block Design	28.95 (10.14)	31.90 (7.97)

Table 2. *Neuropsychological test results in MS patients compared to matched control group.* Results are means (s.d.).

	MS patients (n = 20)	*Controls (n = 20)*
Trail Making A	56.00 (24.95)	32.85 (12.16)§
Trail Making B	118.55 (65.25)	73.20 (25.91)‡
SDMT	34.80 (11.74)	48.80 (10.90)§
Recurring Figures	33.00 (9.12)	40.95 (9.80)§
Visual Gestalt		
Immediate	4.30 (3.97)	2.80 (3.01)
Learning	6.00 (7.38)	3.70 (5.50)
Retention	5.25 (4.87)	5.40 (5.05)
Story Recall	7.50 (2.44)	10.85 (3.04)§
AVLT		
Learning Trail 1	5.30 (1.52)	6.05 (1.39)
Learning Trail 2	7.35 (1.66)	9.05 (1.57)¶
Learning Trail 3	9.35 (2.25)	10.80 (1.76)†
Learning Trail 4	10.30 (2.13)	11.65 (1.87)†
Learning Trail 5	11.20 (2.23)	12.35 (1.87)*
AVLT Delayed Recall	9.50 (2.56)	11.30 (2.55)†

SDMT = Symbol Digit Modalities Test; AVLT = Auditory Verbal Learning Test
*$P<0.10$; †$P<0.05$; ‡$P<0.02$; §$P<0.01$; ¶$P<0.005$

scores on the intelligence subtests. Taken as a group, the MS patients showed relatively moderate physical disability, and on intelligence tests cognitive function was found to be normal and intact.

Evaluation on neuropsychological status showed that the MS group had a lower ranking level in tests assessing attention, information processing speed, visual recognition memory, immediate logical verbal memory, and learning and consolidation of verbal memory. In the 'Auditive Verbal Learning Test', it seemed that the MS group had the same point of origin on the first trial as the control group but did not reach the same level of consolidation. No significant differences were seen in Visual Gestalt Test, a memory test with logical geometrical figures. The *P* values are given in the Table. In terms of groups, it was seen that the MS patients had slight and moderate cognitive impairment compared with controls without CNS disorders.

The ophthalmological examinations showed that all 20 patients were able to read and see the material used in the psychological tests. Analyses of the variance within the MS group

Table 3. *Differences in non-verbal test performance within the MS patient group according to optic disc pathology.* Results are means (s.d.).

	Normal/slight abnormality (n = 10)	*Pathological (n = 10)*
Picture Arrangement	13.20 (5.88)	8.80 (5.73)
Block Design	32.10 (7.75)	25.80 (11.61)
Trail Making A	52.90 (24.93)	59.10 (25.92)
Trail Making B	98.00 (45.67)	139.10 (77.22)
SDMT	39.50 (9.80)	30.10 (12.06)
Recurring Figures	33.90 (10.81)	32.10 (7.53)
Disability Scale Score	3.10 (1.52)	3.50 (0.52)
Mean Age	37.90 (4.74)	39.50 (6.05)

SDMT = Symbol Digit Modalities Test

Table 4. *Differences in non-verbal test performance within the MS patient group according to colour vision*. Results are means (s.d.).

	Normal (n = 11)	*Pathological (n = 9)*
Picture Arrangement	14.18 (4.19)	7.11 (5.92)†
Block Design	32.81 (7.73)	24.22 (11.12)*
Trail Making A	50.90 (23.85)	62.22 (26.23)
Trail Making B	92.90 (44.58)	149.88 (74.95)
SDMT	38.45 (10.45)	30.33 (12.23)
Recurring Figures	34.00 (10.11)	31.77 (8.15)
Visual Gestalt		
I Immediate	3.27 (3.06)	5.55 (4.74)
L Learning	3.36 (3.72)	9.22 (9.52)
Retention	4.18 (4.83)	6.55 (4.87)
Disability Scale Score	3.27 (1.48)	3.33 (0.50)
Mean Age	38.00 (4.64)	39.55 (6.30)

SDMT = Symbol Digit Modalities Test
*$P<0.05$; $^{\dagger}P<0.01$

were carried out for optic discs, colour vision and field defects. For each analysis the MS patients were divided into two groups, one presenting normal findings in the ophthalmological dimension and the other presenting pathological findings.

Table 3 shows a sample of the analyses of the neuropsychological results obtained in the MS group. A small sample is given of the mean scores with standard deviation distribution for the two subgroups. It can be seen that the subgroup presenting pathological findings in the optic disc showed a tendency towards a lower level of performance in the tests requiring visual information processing, but on the rank sum test no significant differences were found.

Nine patients were found to have reduced colour vision. The tests requiring visual perception are listed in Table 4. It is seen that the performance of the group with reduced colour vision has a lower ranking level in these tests than the group with normal colour vision. Significant differences were found in only two intelligence subtests, namely Picture Arrangement and Block Design. The *P* values are given in the Table.

The same trends were not present in the verbal tests and neither was there a significant difference for mean age or disability status score between the groups.

The tendency towards lower performance level in all the tests in the group with poor colour vision makes it difficult to disregard it as a coincidence, though the result is not free of ambiguity due to the small number of patients involved, and because eight of the patients in question had both reduced colour vision and visual field defects.

Colour vision influences distinctness in picture formation and perhaps also object identification. This probably explains the high *P* values seen in the two tests requiring quality in information processing.

Twelve patients were found to have distinct defects in their visual fields. The performance of the subgroup with pathological findings was at a significantly lower ranking level in Trail Making A and B and in all three sections of the Visual Gestalt Test (Table 5). The Table also shows that the group presenting pathological findings generally had a lower performance level than the group without visual field defects. No significant differences were found in verbal intelligence tests and neither was there a tendency towards a lower performance level in the verbal memory tests. This study has confirmed the hypothesis that MS can cause reduced speed in information processing parallel with the presence of defects in the visual fields.

Table 5. *Differences in non-verbal test performance within the MS patient group according to visual fields*. Results are means (s.d.).

	Normal/slight defect (n = *8)*	*Pathological (*n = *12)*
Picture Arrangement	14.00 (5.73)	9.00 (5.67)
Block Design	32.50 (8.99)	26.58 (10.52)
Trail Making A	41.50 (14.25)	65.66 (26.29)*
Trail Making B	84.87 (49.61)	141.00 (66.42)*
SDMT	40.50 (11.33)	31.00 (10.80)
Recurring Figures	35.00 (10.94)	31.66 (7.91)
Visual Gestalt		
Immediate	3.12 (4.01)	5.08 (3.91)*
Learning	3.75 (6.51)	7.50 (7.79)†
Retention	3.25 (3.77)	6.58 (5.21)*
Disability Scale Score	3.00 (1.41)	3.50 (0.90)
Mean Age	37.62 (4.92)	39.41 (5.72)

SDMT = Symbol Digit Modalities Test
$^*P<0.05$; $^\dagger P<0.02$

Loss of portions of the central visual field may particularly impair the acquisition of visual information.[16] This indicates that visual field defects have a negative effect on performance in the tests requiring vision. This should be kept in mind when evaluating test results.

Conclusions

The aim of this pilot study was to obtain information on the impact of specific primary visual defects on neuropsychological test results. A high frequency of permanent specific primary visual defects was found in our patient group. Low quality in picture formation, reduced speed in information processing and impaired visual information acquisition tended to be correlated with reduced colour vision and visual field defects.

It is our conclusion that these are factors that should be taken into account when assessing and analysing the results of neuropsychological tests requiring vision.

Acknowledgements—This work was supported by Fonden for Scleroseramte på Fyn and the Danish Multiple Sclerosis Society. We wish to thank Jesper Boldsen, PhD, for assisting with the statistical analyses.

References

1 Bogousslavsky, J. M. D., Fox, A. J., Carey, L. S., Vinitshi, S., Bass, B. *et al.* (1986): Correlates of brainstem oculomotor disorders in multiple sclerosis. *Arch. Neurol.* **43**, 460–463.
2 Galvin, R. J., Heron, J. R. & Regan, D. (1977): Subclinical optic neuropathy in multiple sclerosis. *Arch. Neurol.* **34**, 666–670.
3 Jacobs, L., Kinkel, P. R. & Kinkel, W. R. (1986): Silent brain lesions in patients with isolated idiopathic optic neuritis. *Arch. Neurol.* **46**, 452–455.
4 Meinberg, O., Flammer, J. & Ludin, H-P. (1982): Subclinical visual field defects in multiple sclerosis. *J. Neurol.* **227**, 125–133.
5 Meienberg, O., Müri, R. & Rabineau, P. A. (1986): Clinical and oculographic examination of saccadic eye movements in diagnose of multiple sclerosis. *Arch. Neurol.* **43**, 438–443.

6 Menabue, R., Nichelly, P. & Bellei, S. (1986): Exposure times for colour discrimination in the parafoveal field: a new procedure to detect subtle visual dysfunction in multiple sclerosis patients. *J. Neurol. Neurosurg. Psychiatry* **49**, 400–404.
7 Sanders, A. E. C. M., Volkers, A. C. W., Van der Poel & Van Lith, G. H. (1986): Estimation of visual function after optic neuritis: a comparison of clinical tests. *Br. J. Ophthalmol.* **70**, 918–924.
8 Graff-Radford, N. R. & Rizzo, M. (1987): Neglect in a patient with multiple sclerosis. *Eur. Neurol.* **26**, 100–103.
9 Enoch, J. M., Campos, E. C. & Bedell, H. E. (1979): Visual resolution in a patient exhibiting a visual fatigue or saturation-like effect. Probably multiple sclerosis. *Arch. Ophthalmol.* **97**, 76–78.
10 Hess, R. F. (1983): Contrast vision and optic neuritis: neural blurring. *J. Neurol. Neurosurg. Psychiatry* **46**, 1023–1030.
11 Plant, G. T. & Hess, R. F. (1985): Temporal frequency discrimination in optic neuritis and multiple sclerosis. *Brain* **108**, 647–676.
12 Celesia, G. G., Kaufman, D. & Cone, S. B. (1986): MS: Simultaneous recording of pattern electroretinography and visual evoked potentials in multiple sclerosis. *Arch. Neurol.* **43**, 1247–1252.
13 Galvin, R. J., Regan, D. & Heron, J. R. (1976): Impaired temporal resolution of vision after acute retrobulbar neuritis. *Brain* **99**, 255–268.
14 Regan, D., Milner, B. A. & Heron, J. R. (1976): Delayed visual perception and delayed visual evoked potentials in the spinal form of multiple sclerosis and in retrobulbar neuritis. *Brain* **99**, 43–66.
15 Caine, E. D., Bamford, K. A., Shiffer, R. B., Shoulson, J. & Sanford, L. (1986): A controlled neuropsychological comparison of Huntington's disease and multiple sclerosis. *Arch. Neurol.* **43**, 249–254.
16 Zihl, J. & Wohlfarth-Englert, A. (1986): The influence of visual field disorders on visual identification tasks. *Eur. Arch. Psychiatry Neurol. Sci.* **236**, 61–64.

V

MENTAL DISORDERS

11

SEVERELY THREATENING EVENTS AND MARKED LIFE DIFFICULTIES PRECEDING ONSET OR EXACERBATION OF MULTIPLE SCLEROSIS

Igor Grant*, George W. Brown†, Tirril Harris†, W. Ian McDonald‡, Thomas Patterson*, and Michael R. Trimble‡

**San Diego V. A. Medical Center and Department of Psychiatry, University of California (San Diego) School of Medicine, La Jolla, USA;*
†Bedford and Royal Holloway Colleges, University of London; and
‡Institute of Neurology, National Hospitals, Queen Square and Maida Vale, London

Summary

We obtained information on stressful life circumstances, using the Life Events and Difficulties Schedule (LEDS) from 39 patients with early multiple sclerosis (MS) and 40 matched non-patient volunteers. The proportion of MS patients who experienced marked life adversity in the year prior to onset of symptoms was significantly higher than for non-patients in the year before interview (77% *vs* 35%). The excess in marked life stress was most evident in the 6 months before onset. Such stressors might explain the timing of symptom exacerbation for some patients with MS, perhaps by perturbing an already unstable neuro-immunological system.

Introduction

There has been speculation that stressful life circumstances can influence onset and exacerbation of symptoms of multiple sclerosis virtually from the time the disease was first described in the middle of the last century. The biograpy of Augustus d'Este raises the question whether emotional arousal over the death of a close relative might have been related to the abrupt beginning of his ophthalmological symptoms.[1] In 1868 Charcot, who first delineated MS as we know it today, commented that grief, worry, and adverse changes

This chapter is a reprint of the article by the same authors and with the same title which appeared in 1989 in the *Journal of Neurology, Neurosurgery, and Psychiatry* **52**, 8–13. Data presented here were also reviewed in part in our chapter in the volume *Life Events and Illness* edited by G. W. Brown and T. O. Harris (The Guilford Press, New York, 1989).

in social circumstances might be causally linked to disease onset,[2] and Moxon's 1873 case report notes a possible association between disease onset and the discovery by his patient of her husband in bed with another woman.[3]

Several American studies, influenced by psychoanalytic theory, suggested that stress could produce cerebrovascular alterations which might be aetiologically related to plaque formation.[4] Others asserted that patients with MS had neurotic conflicts between dominance and submission which expressed themselves as neurological symptoms,[5–7] or that such patients could develop the disorder in the context of protracted emotional arousal,[8] particularly anger,[9] or circumstances which posed a threat to the patient's 'security system'.[10] Engel and associates believed that patients who were vulnerable to multiple sclerosis developed it when their life circumstances caused emotional conflict resulting in the 'giving up–given up complex'.[11]

Provocative as these studies were, their lack of comparison groups left their speculation open to serious question. The first controlled study appears to have been that of Pratt.[12] While noting certain individual patients in whom emotional upheavals seemed to precede exacerbation of symptoms, Pratt did not find a statistically significant difference between MS patients and a non-MS neurological comparison group in their experience of life events. Another large controlled study found that MS patients tended to report more serious interpersonal difficulties prior to onset than did controls, but the magnitude of the difference (19% of MS patients as compared to 12% of controls) left the practical importance of this finding open to question.[13]

Two controlled studies which were reported in the 1980s found significant associations between life events and MS symptomatology. The first compared 100 MS patients with 73 neurological and rheumatological patients.[14] In the two years prior to onset of disease MS patients reported three times as many life events; furthermore, more of the MS patients considered themselves to be subjected to unusual stresses during that period (79% of MS *vs* 54% of controls).

The Denver group of investigators gathered data on life events every 4 months for an average of 20 months from 55 patients with relapsing–remitting MS.[15] Patients who reported significant negative or uncontrollable events were 3.7 times as likely to have an exacerbation as those free of such events.

In sum, despite a wealth of anecdotal evidence suggesting an association between life stresses and exacerbation of MS, the results of controlled studies have been distinctly mixed. We now report on a cohort of MS patients examined at the National Hospital, Queen Square, and compare the experience of our patients to those of matched non-patients using an improved life events method—the Bedford College Life Events and Difficulties Schedule (LEDS)—a technique which has been applied successfully in research into other disorders but not, until the present time, with MS.

Methods

Subjects

Multiple sclerosis group. These patients ($n = 39$) were recent referrals to consultant neurologists at the National Hospitals, Queen Square, and Maida Vale. The median time between symptom onset and entry into the study was two years with a range of 1 to 54 months. Thirty-three of these patients also participated in a related neuropsychological study of deficient learning and memory in early MS, the results of which have already been reported.[16]

There were 10 men and 29 women (originally there were 30 women, but one was excluded because the diagnosis of probable MS turned out to be incorrect). Average age was

35.6 ± 9.0 years. Most (85%) were middle class as defined by points 1–22 on the Hope-Goldthorpe scale.[17] Of these 39 patients, 32 were married and 27 had children. At the time the patients were recruited the diagnostic requirement was that patients must qualify either for probable or definite MS. At the time of this writing, however, all 'probable' patients have had further neurological assessment and all now qualify as definite MS either on clinical grounds or based on laboratory-supported data.[17] At the time of examination 25 of the patients were undergoing diagnostic evaluations as inpatients, and the remaining 14 attended as outpatients. The mean disability score, based on the Kurtzke Expanded Disability Status Scale, was 2.2 (range 1.0–6.5) at time of interview. Although virtually all patients experienced some transient symptoms previously, 23 had their first medically documented episode at the time of this study, while the remaining 16 had relapses. At time of interview 16 patients knew their diagnosis while 23 did not.

Healthy comparison group. Because the authors were engaged in concurrent epidemiological studies of healthy volunteers using the same measures it was possible to recruit non-patients, matched to the MS patients on a case by case basis for age, sex, marital status, and socioeconomic position. The non-patient group consisted of 10 men and 30 women (one additional woman was matched to the patient who was subsequently withdrawn), of whom 28 were married, and 23 had children. Their mean age was 35.7 ± 9.7 years. Based on a rating of 1–22 on the Hope-Goldthorpe scale, 80 percent of this group was middle class.

Life Events Interviews

Three of the four controlled studies reviewed above may have suffered from methodological inadequacies in the gathering of life events information, and these inadequacies could, in part, explain disparate results. One of the studies[14] obtained information on the basis of a self-report check list whose validity increasingly is subject to question.[19–21] The other two performed interviews, but these were idiosyncratic to the specific projects, and hence we have no data on reliability.

The Life Events and Difficulties Schedule (LEDS) developed by Brown and associates has received increasing international recognition as a valid and reliable approach for ascertaining life events, difficulties, and important sources of social support.[19] For this reason, it appeared to represent an advance in the current research. The LEDS consists of a semi-structured interview which probes systematically for the occurrence of life events and difficulties in a comprehensive fashion, covering many different areas. In this project the interviewers received training by the Bedford College team to assure consistency in data gathering. Each interview took approximately 2 hours to complete. In the case of MS patients data on life circumstances were gathered for the year preceding onset of major symptoms. For non-patients, the interview concentrated on information in the year preceding interview. This means that patients were reporting on events which occurred 2 to 3 years prior to the interview while non-patients were recollecting the past year. While this difference in recall length between patients and controls is not ideal, the literature suggests that, if anything, the number of events recalled tends to drop off with length of recall period.[22] Thus, bias in this study would be in the direction against our hypothesis, reducing the number of events reported by patients, and increasing those reported by controls.

Analysis of LEDS information

Information on life circumstances obtained from the LEDS was grouped into two categories: events, and difficulties. Events were happenings occurring at relatively discrete points in time, while difficulties represented life circumstances which went on for 4 weeks or more. Difficulties might begin with a discrete event or might develop more insidiously.

A commonly acknowledged limitation in life events research comes from the appreciation that people can vary widely as to the subjective 'stressfulness' rating which they might attach to a particular happening. For this reason, Brown and Harris[19,23,24] have argued that it is important to supplement subjective ratings with *contextual* ratings.

Contextual ratings

Contextual ratings are performed by the research team after it has heard a precis of a particular subject's situation, life events, and difficulties. Using a set of decision rules that have evolved as part of the LEDS instrument, and by the frequent reference to an extensive dictionary of events and difficulties which have been gathered over several thousand interviews, the investigators can make a judgement as to whether a reported happening should be considered a true event or difficulty (rather than simply a trivial incident, of insufficient importance to include in data analysis), and, if so, what ratings to give to relevant dimensions such as independence, focus, and threat. The threshold for including incidents in data analysis was deliberately set high in terms of their likelihood of arousing a strong positive or negative emotion.[24] Some examples of events which might have been counted in earlier studies, but which were eliminated by our threshold are: patient's husband gives notice to his employer that he is quitting his job, something which the family has planned; death of a patient's grandmother abroad (patient had not seen the grandmother for many years); a patient's son applying to University; a patient's sister having a planned abortion.

Ratings of events

Once an event was included in data analysis, the investigators rated the degree of '*threat*' it posed to the person's security, relationships, future, or some other important aspect of his life. A 4-point scale was used, with level 1 indicating a very severe threat, level 2 moderately severe, level 3 moderate to mild, level 4 mild to minimal. The probable duration of threat was also rated as *short-term* if it was concluded that the major impact of the event had dissipated within 48 hours, or *long-term* if the probable effect was going to be more long-lasting. An example with high short-term threat but little long-term threat would be a parent receiving news that a child was involved in a road accident and was now at a casualty department (threat level = 1, short-term); when the parents arrive at casualty they discover that the child is perfectly fine, simply having a few scratches (long-term threat = 4). On the other hand, if the same parents discover that the child had indeed suffered a cerebral haemorrhage, then the long-term threat would remain severe (level 1). A further variation on the same event might be that the parents were told by the school that their child suffered a minor knock on the head while playing football and seemed perfectly fine (short-term threat = 3); within the next two days the child developed severe headaches, became unconscious, and was found to have an intracranial bleed (long-term threat = 1).

Events were also rated as to *focus*. A rating of *self*-focus (identical to 'subject focus' of Brown & Harris) indicates that the event occurred to the subject directly, or, if it occurred to another important individual in the person's life the subject was, nevertheless, directly involved in some aspect of that happening. Examples of events which would receive self-focus include being sacked, or one's husband being sacked if that circumstance is likely to produce financial hardship on the family. On the other hand, hearing that one's mother has cancer would receive a focus rating of *other* unless the subject was somehow intimately involved in the hospital consultations or immediate caring of the mother.

Events were also classified on the basis that they might conceivably be related to, or even be a product of the MS. For example, a patient who feels unsteady and has blurred vision might have an automobile accident. It would not be appropriate to consider such an event in any causal analysis exploring the influence of events upon the disease. In the results presented, such 'illness-related' events were excluded.

Ratings of difficulty level

Those ongoing life happenings which are more appropriately considered difficulties were also rated as to level of severity using a 6-point scale, in which level 1 represented extreme, hardly tolerable circumstances, whilst difficulties of level 6 were rather minor.

Illness-related difficulties (ie those that might be products of MS or some other medical problem) were not included in the data analyses described below.

Severe events and marked difficulties

Previous research has indicated that of all events, those which pose substantial long-term threat to the person directly are most likely to be associated with medical and psychiatric disorders.[19,26–28] For the purposes of this study, we followed the convention established by Brown and Harris[18] which defined *severely threatening events* as those which received a contextual rating on long-term threat of level 1, or any level 2 event which had a self focus (level 1 events could have either self or other focus).

Marked difficulties were those which received contextual severity ratings at levels 1, 2 or 3. Difficulties rated 4–6 were termed mild difficulties.

Finally, a subject was classified as experiencing a *marked adversity* if he or she reported either a severely threatening event and/or a marked difficulty (as defined above) during the period in question.

Results

Marked adversity

In the 6 months preceding onset, 30 of the 39 MS patients (77%) experienced marked life adversity as defined above. Among non-patients 14 of 40 (35%) reported marked adversity in the 6 months preceding interview. The difference in proportions is highly significant ($\chi^2 = 14.08$, $P < 0.001$). Examples of marked adversity are shown in the Table.

Severely threatening events

Turning to the components of marked adversity which distinguished patients from non-patients, we found that 24 of 39 MS patients (62%) reported a severely threatening event, as compared to 6 of 40 controls (15%) ($\chi^2 = 18.02$, $P < 0.001$). There was no specific category of event (eg, health change in a significant other person; social role change; finances; interpersonal; miscellaneous crises) which accounted for this disproportion. Rather, severe events were scattered throughout all of these content areas.

Marked difficulties

Patients with MS also experienced more marked difficulties in the 6 months prior to onset than did the controls in the 6 months before interview. In this instance, 19/39 patients

Table 1. *Examples of classes of marked adversity*. 'Marked adversity' includes severely threatening events and/or marked difficulties (see Methods)

Class of adversity	*Example*	*Number of MS patients reporting this class of adversity*
Conflicts or prolonged separations involving spouse (or lover), other close family member, or 'confidant'	Example 1: Husband discovers patient is having affair Example 2: Chronic marital friction; couple barely speaks to each other for 9 months Example 3: Son, the patient's closest 'confidant', leaves the area	19
Major illness or death involving spouse (or lover), other close family member, or 'confidant'	Example 1: Patient looks after dependent son with spina bifida; gets little help Example 2: Discovers illicit pregnancy of daughter when it ends in abortion Example 3: Mother makes suicide attempt Example 4: Mother discovered to have cancer	9
Major job-related problems	Example 1: Husband unexpectedly gets redundancy notice; family has little money, and there is no immediate prospect of another job Example 2: Patient is redeployed against her will	5
Interpersonal conflicts with neighbours, landlord, acquaintances, etc. . . .	Example 1: neighbours have frequent noisy and boisterous drinking—frequent confrontations to point patient decides on moving Example 2: Co-worker tries to seduce patient's wife	5
Housing problems	Example 1: patient and husband live in cramped flat shared by mother-in-law. Little privacy. No washing machine	2
Severe financial problems	Patient works long hours without vacation to support husband and unemployed daughter. Every month has trouble making ends meet	1
Other crises or misadventures	Example 1: Patient mugged while walking in neighbourhood. Sustains minor injuries, loses purse with papers and 20 pounds, feels unsafe in neighbourhood Example 2: Driving from party patient is breathalyzed; later fined and loses licence for 1 year (needed for sales job)	3

(49%) *vs* 8/40 controls (20%) experienced marked difficulties throughout the 6 months preceding onset.

Significantly more patients than controls experienced marital difficulties (19/39 [49%] *vs* 4/40 [10%]; $\chi^2 = 9.78$, $P < 0.01$) and difficulties with parents or siblings (13/39 [33%] *vs* 3/40 [8%]; $\chi^2 = 6.24$, $P < 0.02$). Interestingly, somewhat more control subjects reported difficulties with housing (11/40, 28%) compared to MS patients (3/39, 8%; $\chi^2 = 4.58$, $P < 0.05$). There were no other areas of difficulty which differentiated patients from controls.

Timing of events in the year preceding onset

Figure 1 shows the proportion of MS patients and controls reporting a severe life event during each bi-monthly period in the year preceding onset of symptomatology (or the year preceding interview for controls). In the period 7–12 months before onset (interview for controls) approximately 10–15% of subjects in each group experienced a severely threatening event. This rate remained approximately the same for controls right up to the time of interview. In contrast, at 5–6 months prior to onset the proportion of MS patients reporting severe events increased, with more than a third experiencing such an event in the 2 months prior to onset.

The specificity of this finding is underscored by Fig. 2, which shows the occurrence of non-severe events over the same 12-month period. There are no systematic differences between patients and controls in their experience of such events.

Marked adversity in relation to disability and awareness of diagnosis

Since it is possible that environmental stress might have different importance in the precipitation of relapses *vs* initial episodes, we compared the distribution of marked adversity between those experiencing their first medically documented episode ($n = 23$) and

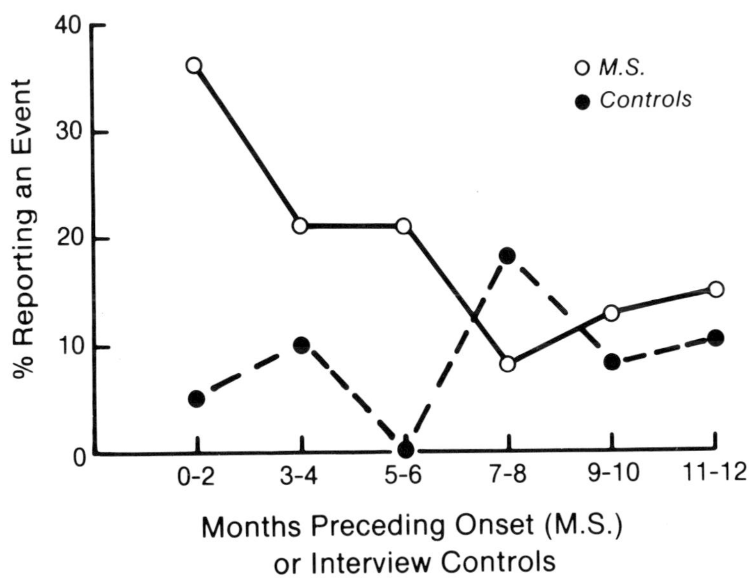

Fig. 1. *Report of severely threatening life events by MS patients (*n = 39*) and controls (*n = 40*)*

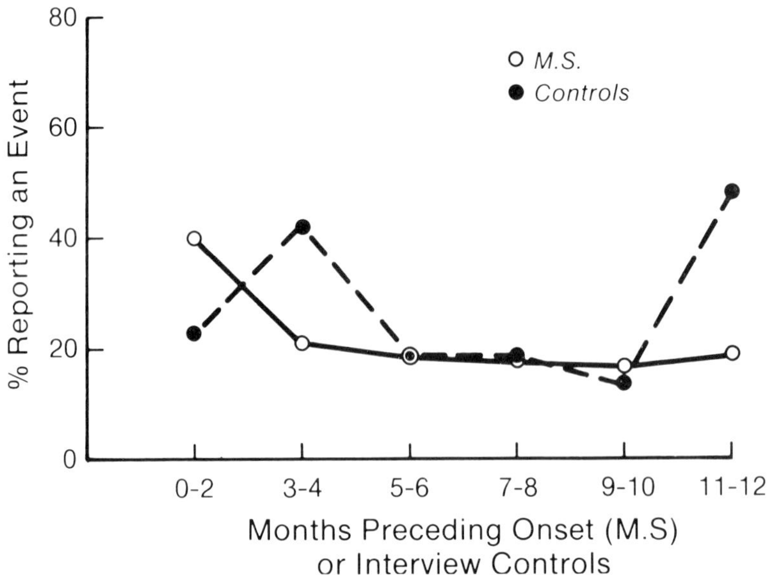

Fig. 2. *Report of less threatening events by MS patients (*n = *39) and controls (*n = *40)*

those with relapses (*n* = 16). Eighteen of 23 first episode cases and 12 of 16 relapsing cases reported marked adversity. Similarly, there was no significant difference in proportion of those reporting marked adversity between patients who knew *versus* those who were unaware of their diagnosis (13/16 *vs* 17/23). There was no systematic association between Kurtzke Disability Scale rating at interview and report of marked adversity. The mean Kurtzke score for those with adversity was 2.1 (range 1.0–6.5) and for those without adversity, 2.3 (range 1.0–4.0).

Discussion

In a retrospective study of patients with relatively recent onset of MS we found that almost three-quarters of these patients experienced a marked adversity in their lives in the 6 months prior to the onset of symptomatology. Only 35% of a non-patient group matched for age, sex, marital status, and social position experienced such adversities. MS patients reported more discrete events of a severely threatening nature, and also somewhat greater levels of ongoing marked life difficulties. While there were no specific classes of events which distinguished patients from controls, longstanding difficulties which seemed to occur more often among patients included concerns about spouse and blood relatives. Some of these concerns involved interpersonal conflict with these important other people, while in other instances such concerns revolved around major health changes affecting such relatives.

While our results fit well with those reported from Alberta[14] and Colorado[15], they are at variance with Antonovsky's survey of MS patients in Israel[13] and also with the conclusions reached by Pratt in another British study conducted some 30 years earlier.[12] While methodological differences could easily explain our disagreement with Antonovsky *et al.*[13] (they questioned their subjects concerning a limited number of life events which could have occurred as much as twenty years previously), the inconsistency with Pratt is more difficult to explain.

It may be, of course, that by using a non-standard interview method Pratt might have failed to question both patients and medical controls sufficiently thoroughly; further, the period of retrospective distortion and forgetting was much longer in Pratt's study since his typical patient was already moderately disabled.

Since the design of our study was also retrospective, it may be legitimate to question whether vagaries in recall or 'effort after meaning' (ie, patients trying to make sense of their symptoms and trying to find reasons for them) might be confounding factors here. With respect to the problem of forgetting, we feel that our study, albeit retrospective, does represent a distinctive step forward through its use of a well validated and reliable life events method—the LEDS. The comprehensive and systematic probing of life circumstances by a trained interviewer makes it less likely that important happenings will be forgotten. At the same time, the method of contextual rating by the investigative team tends to protect the study against inclusion of trivial or idiosyncratically inflated events and difficulties. The exclusion of illness-related events and difficulties attempts to avoid the sort of circularity that sometimes plagues other life events research—for instance, the inclusion by Warren *et al.*[14] of 'personal illness/injury' as one of the categories of life events can raise questions about what came first—the illness or the event?

We believe that our focus on patients with relatively recent onset of disease is another strength. Our patients were individuals who, by and large, experienced their first major symptoms in the preceding 2 to 3 years. This is a much shorter period for which recall has been attempted than has been true for most other studies. Finally, the fact that a longitudinal analysis of our data suggests an upswing in severely threatening life events in the 6 months prior to onset, while rates remained comparable to controls in an earlier 6 month epoch, suggests that patients were not simply over-reporting. This inference is strengthened by the finding that there were no significant differences in less threatening events and less severe difficulties between patients and controls.

While our study indicates a temporal relationship between marked adversity and MS symptoms, we cannot prove that this relationship is causal. Recent neuro-immunological research does provide evidence, however, that stress can induce alterations in immune status.[29] There is also good evidence for the existence of immunological abnormalities in MS, and that these are important in the pathogenesis of disease.[30] Since the precise way in which the immunological defect in multiple sclerosis leads to tissue damage is uncertain, it is impossible to predict how further alterations induced by stress could initiate or reactivate the disease process. These difficulties notwithstanding, our data, taken with those of other recent investigations, provide evidence for the view that there is a connection between stressful life events and the onset of symptoms or relapse in MS.

Acknowledgements—Support for this work was provided by the Medical Research Service of the Veterans Administration and by the Foundations Fund for Research in Psychiatry. The authors are indebted to Dr. P. C. Gautier-Smith for his enthusiastic support of this study, and particularly, his willingness to identify patients who might be suitable as research subjects. Professors John Marshall, J. Newsom-Davis, and P. K. Thomas were also helpful in allowing us access to patients, as were Drs R. W. Ross Russell, J. A. Morgan-Hughes, P. Rudge, A. N. Gale, R. Clifford Jones, A. J. Lees, P. Bradbury, and E. Byrne. Ms Marge Zeitsman assisted in scheduling some of our patients. The authors are grateful to Michelle Page for preparing the manuscript.

References

1 Firth, D. (1948): *The case of Augustus d'Este.* Cambridge: Cambridge University Press.
2 Charcot, J. M. (1868): Lectures on the diseases of the nervous system delivered at La Salpetriere. London: New Sydenham Society, 1877, translated by G. Sigerson.

3 Moxon, W. (1873): Case of insular sclerosis of brain and spinal cord. *Lancet*: 236.
4 Jelliffe, S. E. (1921): Multiple sclerosis and psychoanalysis. *Am. J. Med. Sci.* **161**, 666–675.
5 Langworthy, O. R., Kolb, L. C. & Androp, S. (1941): Disturbances of behavior in patients with disseminated sclerosis. *Am. J. Psychiatry* **98**, 243–249.
6 Langworthy, O. R. (1948): Relation of personality problems to onset and progress of multiple sclerosis. *Arch. Neurol. Psychiatry* **59**, 13–28.
7 Langworthy, O. R. (1950): A survey of the maladjustment problems in multiple sclerosis and the possibilities of psychotherapy. *Proceedings of the Association for Research in Nervous and Mental Diseases* **28**, 598–611.
8 Braceland, F. J. & Giffin, M. E. (1950): The mental changes associated with multiple sclerosis (an interim report). *Proceedings of the Association for Research in Nervous and Mental Diseases* **28**, 450–455.
9 Grinker, R. R., Ham, G. C. & Robbins, F. P. (1950): Some psychodynamic factors in multiple sclerosis. *Proceedings of the Association for Research in Nervous and Mental Diseases* **28**, 456–460.
10 Philippopoulos, G. S., Wittkower, E. D. & Cousineau, A. (1958): The etiologic significance of emotional factors in onset and exacerbations of multiple sclerosis. *Psychosom. Med.* **20**, 458–474.
11 Mei-Tal, V., Meyerowitz, S. & Engel, G. L. (1970): The role of psychological process in a somatic disorder: multiple sclerosis. *Psychosom. Med.* **32**, 67–86.
12 Pratt, R. T. C. (1951): An investigation of the psychiatric aspects of disseminated sclerosis. *J. Neurol. Neurosurg. Psychiatry* **14**, 326–336.
13 Antonovsky, A., Leibowitz, U., Medalie, J. M., Smith, H. A., Halpern, L. & Alter, M. (1968): Reappraisal of possible etiologic factors in multiple sclerosis. *Am. J. Public Health* **58**, 836–848.
14 Warren, S., Greenhill, S. & Warren, K. G. (1982): Emotional stress and the development of multiple sclerosis: case-control evidence of a relationship. *J. Chronic Dis.* **35**, 821–831.
15 Franklin, G. M., Nelson, L. M., Heaton, R. K., Burks, J. S., & Thompson, D. S. Stress and its relationship to acute exacerbations in multiple sclerosis. *J. Neurol. Rehab.* (1988): **2**: 7–11.
16 Grant, I., McDonald, W. I., Trimble, M. R., Smith, E. & Reed, R. (1984): Deficient learning and memory in early and middle phases of multiple sclerosis. *J. Neurol. Neurosurg. Psychiatry* **47**, 250–255.
17 Goldthorpe, J. H. & Hope, K. (1974): *The social grading of occupations: a new approach and scale*. London: Oxford University Press.
18 Poser, C. M., Paty, D. W., Scheinberg, L., McDonald, W. I., Davis, F. A., Ebers, G. C., Johnson, K. P., Sibley, W. A., Silberberg, D. H. & Tourtellotte, W. W. (1983): New diagnostic criteria for multiple sclerosis: guidelines for research protocols. *Ann. Neurol.* **13**, 227–336.
19 Brown, G. W. & Harris, T. (1978): *Social origins of depression: a study of psychiatric disorders in women*. London: Tavistock, 1978.
20 Grant, I., Yager, J., Sweetwood, H. L. & Olshen, R. (1982): Life events and symptoms. Fourier analysis of time series from a three-year prospective inquiry. *Arch. Gen. Psychiatry* **39**, 598–605.
21 Grant, I., Patterson, T. L., Olshen, R. & Yager, J.(1987): Life events do not predict symptoms: symptoms predict symptoms. *J. Behav. Med.* **10**, 231–241.
22 Nielson, E., Brown, G. W. & Marmot, M. (1988): Myocardial infarction. In *Life events and illness*, eds G. W. Brown & T. O. Harris. New York: Guilford Press.
23 Brown, G. W. (1974): Meaning, measurement, and stress of life events. In *Stressful life events: their nature and effects*, eds B. S. Dohrewend & B. P. Dohrewend. New York: John Wiley.
24 Brown, G. W. (1988): Life events and measurement. In *Life events and illness*, eds G. W. Brown & T. O. Harris. New York: Guilford Press.
25 Brown, G. W. & Birley, J. (1968): Crises and life changes and the onset of schizophrenia. *J. Health Soc. Behav.* **9**, 203–214.
26 Craig, T. K. J. & Brown, G. W. (1988): Goal frustration and life events in the aetiology of painful gastrointestinal disorder. In *Life events and illness*, eds G. W. Brown & T. O. Harris. New York: Guilford Press.
27 Creed, F. (1981): Life events and appendicectomy. *Lancet* **1**, 381–385.

28 Harris, T. O. (1988): Disorders of menstruation. In *Life events and illness*, eds G. W. Brown & T. O. Harris. New York: Guilford Press.
29 Calabrese, J. R., Kling, M. A. & Gold, P. W. (1987): Alterations in immunocompetence during stress, bereavement, and depression: focus on neuroendocrine regulation. *Am. J. Psychiatry* **144**, 1123–1134.
30 Lightman, A., McDonald, W. I., Bird, A. C., Francis, D. A., Hoskins, A., Batchelor, J. R. & Halliday, A. M. (1987): Retinal venous sheathing in optic neuritis: Its significance for the pathogenesis of multiple sclerosis. *Brain* **110**, 405–414.

12

EUPHORIA IN MULTIPLE SCLEROSIS

Peter V. Rabins

The Johns Hopkins University School of Medicine, Meyer 279, 600 N. Wolfe St., Baltimore, MD 21205, USA

Euphoria is an uncommon psychological symptom in multiple sclerosis (MS) and almost always occurs in the setting of diffuse brain disease and dementia. Probably more common but less well studied is the 'eutonia' described more than 50 years ago by Kinnear-Wilson.

Euphoria is probably the most controversial emotional symptom reported in MS. Reports of the prevalence of euphoria range from 0%[1] to more than 80%.[2] Most studies, however, report prevalence rates below 25% and the true prevalence is likely to be even lower. Nonetheless, euphoria is among the symptoms most known to health practitioners.

Charcot mentioned 'foolish laughter without cause' in his original listing of emotional changes seen in MS.[3] In the 1920s several studies focused on this issue and have strongly influenced current views on its high prevalence. Brown & Davis[4] reported it as occurring in 10 of 14 patients with 'mental symptoms' and distinguished between euphoria and mania, suggesting that mania was less common. Cottrell & Wilson[2] identified three different types of elevated mood and noted that other patients had significant emotional lability. They reported that 63% of 100 subjects had some form of euphoria and that 84% had a shift in mood toward increased optimism. Sachs & Freedman,[5] in contrast, reported a 17% rate of explosive laughter and emotional instability. Most recent studies have reported prevalence rates in the range reported by Sachs & Freedman.[5] Surridge,[6] for example, reported a rate of 25.9%. He found no euphoria in patients with muscular dystrophy, thus concluding that it was a specific emotional concomitant of MS. He also noted clinically that many individuals who appeared euphoric described their moods as fluctuating and that many were actually experiencing periods of low mood. Of most importance was his finding that most individuals who were euphoric were demented. He concluded that a relationship which had been suggested by Brown & Davis[4] and Ombredane,[7] that euphoria is a concomitant of cognitive impairment in MS and thus resulted from the extent of brain involvement, was confirmed.

In a recent study of 87 patients with multiple sclerosis,[8] we compared the relationships among a number of variables which measured disease severity and the presence of euphoria as identified by the treating neurologist. We did not distinguish between patients who had the outward expression of euphoria (what Cottrell & Wilson called 'eutonia') and patients who reported the internal mood experience of persistent cheerfulness (what Cottrell & Wilson called 'euphoria sclerotica'). We found that euphoric patients were more likely to have evidence of brain involvement as opposed to involvement of the spinal cord only ($P = 0.006$), were more likely to have enlarged ventricles ($P = 0.04$), to score more poorly on the Mini Mental State Exam,[9] a brief cognitive screening examination ($P = 0.04$), and to be more physically ill ($P = 0.05$) and functionally disabled ($P = 0.01$). Emotional lability, on the other hand, correlated with none of these variables. Thus we concluded like Surridge[6] that euphoria is predominantly the result of structural brain diseases rather than a psychogenic denial of dysfunction and disability.

References

1 Braceland, F. J. & Giffin, M. E. (1950): The mental changes associated with multiple sclerosis (an interim report). *Research Publications: Association for Research in Nervous and Mental Diseases* **28**, 450–455.
2 Cottrell, S. S. & Wilson, S. A. K. (1926): The affective symptomatology of disseminated sclerosis. *J. Neurol. Psychopathol.* **7**, 1–30.
3 Charcot, J. M. (1877): *Lectures on the diseases of the nervous system* (Translated by G. Sigerson). London: New Sydenham Society.
4 Brown, S. & Davis, T. K. (1922): The mental symptoms of multiple sclerosis. *Arch. Neurol. Psychiatry* **7**, 629–634.
5 Sachs, B. & Friedman, E. D. (1922): General symptomatology and differential diagnosis of disseminated sclerosis. *Arch. Neurol. Psychiatry* **7**, 551–560.
6 Surridge, D. (1969): An investigation into some psychiatric aspects of multiple sclerosis. *Br. J. Psychiatry* **115**, 749–764.
7 Ombredane, A. (1929): Sur les troubles mentaux de la sclérose en plaques. Thèse de Paris, cited in Surridge (1969).
8 Rabins, P. V., Brooks, B. R., O'Donnell, P., *et al.* (1986): Structural brain correlates of emotional disorder in multiple sclerosis. *Brain* **109**, 585–587.
9 Folstein, M. F., Folstein, S. E. & McHugh, P. R. (1975): "Mini-mental state": A practical method for grading the cognitive state of patients for the clinician. *J. Psychiatr. Res.* **12**, 189–198.

13

MOOD DISORDER AND MULTIPLE SCLEROSIS

Russell T. Joffe*, Gerard P. Lippert*, Trevor A. Gray†, Gordon Sawa†, and Ziporah Horvath*

**Department of Psychiatry and †Neurology, St. Michael's Hospital, and the University of Toronto, Toronto, Ontario, Canada*

Introduction

Multiple sclerosis (MS) is a chronic demyelinating disease of the nervous system which may be progressive and severe. The irregular demyelination of both the central and peripheral nervous systems results in motor, sensory and cognitive impairments of varying degree. In addition, the association of MS with disorders of emotion has been noted since Charcot in 1874. In 1969 Surridge examined the psychiatric status of 108 MS patients under the age of 40 in a partially controlled study.[1] He found that 62% of these patients showed at least mild intellectual deterioration and that 27% were depressed. Surridge concluded that the depression was psychogenic and reactive. He also demonstrated a significant correlation between euphoria and intellectual deterioration which led him to conclude that the euphoria must be a result of damage to the central nervous system.

Whitlock & Siskind compared the incidence of depression in a group of 30 MS patients with a matched control group of patients with other chronic neurological diseases using psychiatric interview and the Beck Depression Inventory.[2] They determined that depression was significantly more common in the MS group than in the control group and, in addition, that more MS patients had suffered episodes of depression in the past than had patients in the control group. Schiffer *et al.*[3] used the Beck Depression Inventory (BDI) and a modified Schedule for Affective Disorders and Schizophrenia to assess current and past depression in two matched groups of MS patients: 15 patients who had predominantly cerebral involvement and 15 whose disease was primarily cerebellar or spinal. They found significantly more depressive episodes in the patients with cerebral involvement than the cerebellar or spinal group but there was no difference in the incidence of current depressive symptomatology or non-affective measures such as degree of disability, duration or pattern of illness or cognitive impairment. They concluded that MS patients with cerebral involvement are more vulnerable to depression and this might possibly be the result of subcortical demyelination.

Dalos *et al.*[4] investigated prospectively the prevalence of depression in 64 MS patients compared to 23 spinal cord injury (SCI) patients using a 28-item subscale of the General Health Questionnaire (GHQ) which was self-administered periodically over the course of a year. Twelve MS patients suffered an exacerbation during the study, nine of whom were also at some point in remission. They found that the MS patients in remission had similar scores to the SCI patients on the depression subscale. Those having an exacerbation, as a group, had a significantly higher score on the depression subscale. McIvor *et al.*[5] studied depression in a group of 120 MS patients whose disease was limited to the spinal cord and who had no history of depression prior to the onset of MS. They determined that in these patients the degree of depression as measured by the BDI was significantly correlated with the absence of remissions in the course of illness, higher age, extent of disability and the perception of lack of support from family and friends. However, these variables did not explain 35% of the variance in the BDI scores and this led them to suggest that other factors might be involved. Schiffer & Babigan,[6] using epidemiological techniques, identified all patients in hospital who had received the diagnosis of MS, temporal lobe epilepsy (TLE) or amyotrophic lateral sclerosis (ALS) and matched them against a register of all psychiatric contacts in that county. They found that a significantly higher proportion of MS patients (62%) than TLE or ALS patients were depressed and that more MS patients had sought psychiatric treatment following the neurological diagnosis.

A number of case reports and studies have also suggested an association between euphoria, mania or hypomania and MS. Surridge found 26% of MS patients to be euphoric and identified three patients who had 'manic–depressive mood swings'.[1] However, he carefully distinguished between hypomania and euphoria on the basis of hyperactivity and flight of ideas and concluded that his euphoric patients were not, in general, hypomanic. Several case reports of patients with coexisting mania and MS have also been published.[7–11] Schiffer *et al.*[12] have investigated the possible association between MS and bipolar disorder in an epidemiological study. Using standard prevalence rates they estimated that they would find 5.4 patients suffering both disorders. However, 10 were identified—a significant excess.

Materials and methods

It can be seen that several studies have consistently supported the association of MS and mood disorders. Although these studies vary in their methodological soundness, none has studied a large group of patients using a standard psychiatric interview and a battery of valid, reliable rating scales. In this study we have carried out a systematic evaluation of the prevalence of mood disorder in a group of patients with well established MS. The Multiple Sclerosis Clinic at St. Michael's Hospital has about 800 registered patients. It is estimated that there are approximately 2500 MS patients in Metro Toronto. During a 6 month period the first 100 patients who attended the clinic for their regular follow-up visit and who gave consent were included in the study. New referrals and patients unable to give informed consent by reason of cognitive impairment were excluded. Of the 100 subjects, 63 were female, 37 were male; the mean age was 42.3 years (s.d. 13.0, range 20–71).

A modified version of the Schedule for Affective Disorders and Shizophrenia-Lifetime Version (SADS-L) was given so as to allow us to make psychiatric diagnoses according to Research Diagnostic Criteria.[13,14] The Criteria were modified so that obtaining professional help for the disorder became the defining criterion rather than functional impairment alone. At the time of interview the following assessment instruments were also completed: the Beck Depression Inventory,[15] the Hamilton Rating Scale for Depression,[16] the Speilberger State Anxiety Inventory,[17] and the Mania Rating Scale.[18] During the MS clinic visit on the day of our assessment, the Kurtzke Disability and Functional Scales were also completed.[19] The Kurtzke Disability Status Scale is a 10 point scale that assesses the overall degree of disability due to MS; a score of 5 indicates that the patient is able to walk unassisted for 200 m and has disability sufficient to impair full daily activities. The Kurtzke Functional scale measures function of various components of the nervous system such as mental, pyramidal, cerebellar and brainstem function. Each subject's case record was carefully reviewed to ascertain the age at which mood symptoms were first noted and to establish any relationship between an episode of mood illness as defined by the SADS-L and the use of corticosteroids. The diagnosis of mood disorder was rejected if all mood episodes were temporally related to periods of steroid use.

Results

The diagnoses according to Research Diagnostic Criteria are shown in Tables 1 and 2. There is some overlap in the diagnoses. We identified 14 subjects with a current diagnosis and 47 with a past diagnosis of major depression. Two of the current depressives and nine of those with a past history of depression were bipolar. The prevalence of minor and intermittent depression, hypomania, generalized anxiety and panic anxiety are also shown. We identified 42 subjects who have a current episode or have had a past episode of major depression and have not been manic or hypomanic; these met the Research Diagnostic Criteria for major depressive disorder. Thirteen subjects had a life-time diagnosis of bipolar disorder which also met the criteria. These were subjects who had a history of both mania or hypomania and depression for which they have sought professional help. Only 28 subjects were free of current or past major psychiatric disorder.

The scores for the mood and disability scales are shown on Tables 3 and 4. The lifetime depression group is equivalent to those with a major depressive disorder. The significant differences noted were that MS patients with no psychiatric diagnosis scored lower than the lifetime depressives on the Beck Depression Inventory, Hamilton Rating Scale for Depression and Speilberger State Anxiety Inventory. The group with no diagnosis also had

Table 1. *Research Diagnostic Criteria diagnoses in MS patients.*

	Current	*Past*
Major depression	14	47
Major depression—bipolar	2	9
Minor depression	1	9
Intermittent depression	1	4
Hypomania	1	2
Generalized anxiety	0	3
Panic anxiety	1	5

Table 2. *Research Diagnostic Criteria lifetime diagnoses in MS patients.*

Major depressive disorder	42
Bipolar disorder	13
Schizophrenia	0
No psychiatric diagnosis	28

Table 3. *Mood and disability scales.* Results are means ± s.d.

	Bipolar (n = *13)*	Lifetime depression (n = *42)*	No diagnosis (n = *28)*
BDI	8.8 ± 4.4	11.6 ± 6.6	6.6 ± 5.5*
HRS-D	6.8 ± 2.6	8.5 ± 4.8	5.6 ± 4.4*
SAS	36.0 ± 13.0	41.0 ± 10.3	33.1 ± 10.2*
MRS	20.1 ± 6.7	24.7 ± 17.4	21.0 ± 12.5
Kurtzke DSS	5.8 ± 1.9	4.6 ± 2.1	5.9 ± 1.6*

*$P < 0.01$ no diagnosis *vs* lifetime depression
BDI = Beck Depression Inventory; HRS-D = Hamilton Rating Scale for Depression; SAS = Speilberger Anxiety Scale; MRS = Mania Rating Scale; Kurtzke DSS = Kurtzke Disability Status Scale

Table 4. *Mood scales: current depression.* Results are means ± s.d.

	Current depression (n = *14)*	Others (n = *86)*
BDI	24.0 ± 10.6*	9.1 ± 6.0
HRS-D	14.5 ± 6.9*	7.4 ± 4.6
SAS	54.2 ± 12.6*	37.2 ± 10.9

*$P < 0.0001$ current depression *vs* all others
For abbreviations see Table 3.

a significantly higher mean Kurtzke Disability status score than did the major depressive group. However, there were no differences between the depressives and the patients with no psychiatric diagnosis on any of the Kurtzke Functional status scales. No significant difference in any mood or functional scale was found between the bipolar group and either the depressives or the group with no diagnosis. We compared the 14 subjects with a current diagnosis of depression with all other subjects and, as would be expected, they scored significantly higher on the mood scales.

We also assessed the degree of correlation between the various scales using Pearson's correlation coefficients. In the whole group, there was a highly significant correlation between the Hamilton and the Beck scores and between the Speilberger and the Beck scores. In addition there was a correlation between the Kurtzke mental function score and both the Beck and Speilberger scales. However, there was no significant relationship between any of the other Kurtzke functional scores and the mood scales.

We evaluated the relationship between the onset of MS symptoms and the occurrence of mood symptoms. These results are shown in Table 5. Of the 42 patients with a lifetime history of major depressive disorder seven were found to have an onset of depression at least 2 years before MS symptoms began and 25 had experienced depression two years or more after the onset of MS symptoms. In the remaining 10 subjects the onset of depression occurred within 2 years of the first MS symptoms. In the group of 13 bipolar subjects, mood illness had preceded MS by at least 2 years in two, the disorders occurred within 2 years of each other in three, and mood symptoms followed MS by more than 2 years in eight.

Table 5. *Onset of mood symptoms and multiple sclerosis.*

	Depression	*Bipolar disorder*
Mood symptoms >2 yrs prior to MS symptoms	7	2
Mood symptoms at approx same time as MS symptoms	10	3
Mood symptoms >2 yrs after onset of MS symptoms	25	8

Table 6. *Family history—MS patients.*

	Current	*Past*
Major depression	3	13
Intermittent depression	2	2
Bipolar disorder	0	1
Generalized anxiety	2	1
Panic disorder	3	0
Schizophrenia	2	0

Table 7. *Family history—MS patients with mood disorder.*

	Lifetime depression (n = 42)	*Bipolar disorder (n = 13)*	*No diagnosis (n = 28)*
Major depression	10	4	2
Bipolar	0	1	0

We were also able to investigate the prevalence of psychiatric disorders in the first degree relatives of the subjects in our study. A modified form of Research Diagnostic Criteria for family history was used to obtain a history of mood disorder, anxiety disorder and schizophrenia in these relatives.[20,21] The psychiatric diagnoses of the first degree relatives of all the subjects are shown in Table 6. We then looked more closely at the prevalence of mood disorder in the relatives of the MS subjects with mood illness. These results are shown in Table 7. Although it appears that there was a higher proportion of MS patients with both lifetime depression and bipolar disorder who had relatives with mood disorder as compared to those with no psychiatric diagnosis, this difference is not significant.

Discussion

Our subjects as a group suffer from moderately severe MS but were not a severely impaired institutionalized group with advanced disease. Nevertheless, our data show that, using strict diagnostic criteria, there is a very high prevalence of both current and lifetime mood disorder in our group of MS patients compared with the general population. We found 14/100 subjects with a current diagnosis of major depression compared to the expected rate of 3–4/100 in the general population as estimated by Boyd & Weissman.[22] Forty-two out of 100 patients met Research Diagnostic Criteria for lifetime major depressive disorder, more than twice the prevalence of about 20/100 estimated by Boyd & Weissman. Our most striking finding is the high lifetime prevalence of bipolar disorder. We identified 13/100 bipolar patients compared to an expected rate of about 1/100. Other studies have suggested an association of mood disorder and MS but have had several methodological limitations. However, our study, in which we have used standardized methodology and a large sample size, provides powerful confirmation of the connection between mood disorder and MS. This relationship is particularly strong with bipolar disorder.

Some of the previous studies have suggested that patients with a greater degree of disability are more likely to experience depression. We have found no direct relationship between degree of disability and mood disorder. In fact, patients with no lifetime psychiatric diagnosis were significantly more disabled than those with lifetime major depression. Our data are not consistent with the observation of Schiffer *et al.*[3] that cerebral rather than cerebellar or spinal MS is more likely to be associated with a history of depression. In our study, patients with lifetime depression were no different from others on mean scores of mental, pyramidal or other aspects of nervous system function. Our findings indicate that in moderately disabled MS patients depression may be an early complication of the disease and related to factors other than physical disability. In addition, our striking finding of the strong association of bipolar disorder and MS cannot be explained as a reaction to physical disability.

When we examined the relationship between the onset of mood symptoms and MS, we found that in most but not all MS patients the mood disorder followed the occurrence of the neurological disorder. This does not establish a causal relationship of course, but it does support other evidence suggesting that mood symptoms result in some way from the MS disease process. Our data on the psychiatric family history of MS patients show that the prevalence of mood disorder in the first degree relatives of these patients is consistent with that reported for the general population. Furthermore, despite the high prevalence of mood illness in the patient group, first degree relatives of MS patients with a history of mood illness as compared to those with no psychiatric diagnosis do not have a significantly higher prevalence of diagnoses of mood disorder. Therefore, mood disorder in MS patients does not appear to conform with the recognizable familial patterns of transmission seen in patients with primary mood disorder.[23]

Conclusion

In a systematic assessment of patients with well established MS, we have found a correlation between mood disorder and MS, an association which is particularly strong for bipolar disorder. This association does not appear to be a reaction to the disability suffered by MS patients nor does the association follow the familial pattern of primary mood disorder. Rather, mood disorder appears more likely to be related to some structural or neurochemical brain lesion resulting from the MS disease process. It is apparent that further research into these possible structural and biochemical correlates of MS and mood disorder is required. More importantly, it is clear that the high prevalence of mood disorder contributes significantly to the morbidity associated with MS. Anecdotal evidence strongly suggests that early recognition and aggressive treatment of mood symptoms in MS is likely to be effective and to improve the quality of life. Further research is necessary to confirm this hypothesis.

References

1 Surridge, D. (1969): An investigation into some aspects of multiple sclerosis. *Br. J. Psychiatry* **115**, 749–764.

2 Whitlock, F. A. & Siskind, M. M. (1980): Depression as a major symptom of multiple sclerosis. *J. Neurol. Neurosurg. Psychiatry* **43**, 861–865.
3 Schiffer, R. B., Caine, E. D. & Bamford, K. A. (1983): Depressive episodes in patients with multiple sclerosis. *Am. J. Psychiatry* **140**, 1498–1500.
4 Dalos, N. P., Rabins, P. V. & Brooks, R. B. (1983): Disease activity and emotional state in multiple sclerosis. *Ann. Neurol.* **13**, 573–577.
5 McIvor, G. P., Riklan, M. & Reznikoff, M. (1984): Depression in multiple sclerosis as a function of length and severity of illness, age, remission and perceived social support. *J. Clin. Psychol.* **40**, 1028–1033.
6 Schiffer, R. B. & Babigan, H. M. (1984): Behavioral disorders in multiple sclerosis, temporal lobe epilepsy and amyotrophic lateral sclerosis: an epidemiological study. *Arch. Neurol.* **41**, 1067–1069.
7 Kellner, C. H., Davenport, Y. & Post, R. M. (1984): Rapidly cycling bipolar disorder and multiple sclerosis. *Am. J. Psychiatry* **141**, 112–113.
8 Paselow, E. D., Deutsch, S. I. & Fieve, R. R. (1981): Coexisting manic symptoms and multiple sclerosis. *Psychosomatics* **22**, 824–825.
9 Mapelli, G. & Ramelli, E. (1981): Manic syndrome associated with multiple sclerosis: secondary mania? *Acta Psychiatr. Belg.* **81**, 337–349.
10 Solomon, J. G. (1978): Multiple sclerosis masquerading as lithium toxicity. *J. Nerv. Ment. Dis.* **166**, 663–665.
11 Kemp, K., Lion, J. R. & Magram, G. Lithium in the treatment of a manic patient with multiple sclerosis: a case report. *Dis. Nerv. Syst.* **38**, 210–211.
12 Schiffer, R. B., Wineman, N. M. & Weitkamp, L. R. (1986): Association between bipolar affective disorder and multiple sclerosis. *Am. J. Psychiatry* **143**, 94–95.
13 Spitzer, R. L. & Endicott, J. (1978): *Schedule for Affective Disorders and Schizophrenia—Lifetime Version (SADS-L).* 3rd ed. New York: Psychiatric Institute.
14 Spitzer, R. L., Endicott, J. & Robins, E. (1978): Research Diagnostic Criteria: rationale and reliability. *Arch. Gen. Psychiatry* **35**, 773–782.
15 Beck, A. T., Ward, C. H. & Mendelson, M. (1961): An inventory for measuring depression. *Arch. Gen. Psychiatry* **4**, 561–571.
16 Hamilton, M. (1960): A rating scale for depression. *J. Neurol. Neurosurg. Psychiatry* **23**, 56–62.
17 Speilberger, C. B., Gorsuch, R. L. & Luschene, R. E. (1970): *STAI manual for the State-Trait Anxiety Inventory.* Palo Alto, CA: Consulting Psychologist Press Inc.
18 Beigel, A., Murphy, D. L. & Bunney, W. E. (1971): The Manic-State Rating Scale: scale construction, reliability and validity. *Arch. Gen. Psychiatry* **25**, 256–262.
19 Kurtzke, J. F. (1961): On the evaluation of disability in multiple sclerosis. *Neurology* **11**, 686–694.
20 Andreasen, N. C., Endicott, J. & Spitzer, R. L. (1977): The family history method using diagnostic criteria. *Arch. Gen. Psychiatry* **34**, 1229–1235.
21 Andreasen, N. C., Rice, J. & Endicott, J. (1986): The family history approach to diagnosis. *Arch. Gen. Psychiatry* **43**, 421–429.
22 Boyd, J. H. & Weissman, N. M. (1982): Epidemiology. In *Handbook of affective disorders*, ed E. S. Paykel, pp 109–125. New York: Guilford Press.
23 Gershon, E. S., Bunney, W. E. & Leckman, J. F. (1976): The inheritance of affective disorders: a review of data hypotheses. *Behav. Genet.* **6**, 227–261.

14

CHARACTERISTICS AND PREDICTORS OF DEPRESSION IN MULTIPLE SCLEROSIS

Sarah L. Minden*, John Orav† and Peter Reich‡

**Division of Psychiatry, Brigham and Women's Hospital, Harvard University; †Department of Biostatistics, Harvard School of Public Health; and ‡Division of Psychiatry, Brigham and Women's Hospital, Harvard University, Boston, USA.*

Summary

We used the Schedule for Affective Disorders, Research Diagnostic Criteria, Family History-Diagnostic Criteria, and Beck Depression Inventory to determine the rates and nature of depression among 50 multiple sclerosis (MS) patients, and to isolate predictors for the occurrence and severity of depressive episodes. Fifty-four percent of patients had major depressions at some time in their lives, according to the Research Diagnostic Criteria, with a significant increase in the rate after the onset of MS symptoms. The MS patients were significantly more depressed than other medical patients described in the literature. Major depressions were associated with exacerbations treated with ACTH or prednisone and a history of major depression both before and after the onset of MS. Depressions were moderately severe and characterized by anger, irritability, worry, and discouragement. Clinical issues in diagnosis and treatment are discussed.

Introduction

For many years researchers have been intrigued with the unusually high rate of depression in multiple sclerosis (MS). Several recent studies using matched controls and standardized instruments have found similar rates of depression, in the range of 27–45%.[1-4] The relationships between depression and exacerbation,[5,6] severity[1-3,6-9] and duration of MS,[1,7,8] cognitive change,[2,9-12] and perceived social support[8] remain unclear.

We conducted this study to look more closely at the kinds of depressive episodes MS patients were experiencing and to see if we could find predictors for those patients who were most at risk for depression.

Methods

Patients

We obtained 50 MS patients by asking every third patient with definite MS[13] who had been seen by the neurology service to participate. All patients were between 20 and 60 years old, were able to enter or leave a wheelchair independently, and were not taking ACTH. There were 19 men and 31 women with a mean age of 40.5 years (s.d. 8.6) and mean education of 14.0 years (s.d. 0.4). Thirty-three patients were married, 11 were single, and six were widowed, separated or divorced. Twenty-nine families had children living at home. Over 60 percent of the patients were in the two highest social classes according to the Hollingshead-Redlich four-factor method of determining socioeconomic status.[14] The demographic characteristics of our sample were similar to a large multi-centre group of 249 patients[15] except that ours contained more professionals ($\chi^2 = 12.18$, df$=4$, $P<0.03$). Seven patients refused to participate because they had no transportation, four were afraid they would become upset, and two felt it would not benefit them.

Measures

We used the Schedule for Affective Disorders and Schizophrenia,[16] a structured interview for assessing the severity of psychiatric symptoms, and then assigned psychiatric diagnoses to the patients according to the Research Diagnostic Criteria.[17,18] We used the Family History-Research Diagnostic Criteria[19,20] to determine if there were affective disorders in first degree relatives. In order not to confuse symptoms of depression with those of MS, we modified the criteria for major depression by replacing fatigue and poor concentration with any two criteria from the list for minor depression except somatic concern. We shortened the criteria for minor depression by simply deleting these three criteria. We subtyped the probable and definite major depressions in the year preceding the study using the Research Diagnostic Criteria.

In interviewing patients we made every effort to ensure that the symptoms they reported were true indicators of depression rather than of MS or of some particular disability, for example a loss of interest in activities as opposed to loss of the physical capacity to perform them. We took the medical and psychiatric histories at separate points in the interview to minimize any tendency for patients to conflate the temporal sequence of these two types of events. Each patient's account was confirmed or amended by interviewing a family member and by reviewing the medical record.

Patients completed the Beck Depression Inventory,[21] with help from a research assistant if they showed clinical evidence of cognitive impairment. No patient was too impaired to be a reliable subject.

Within one week of the psychiatric evaluation, a senior neurologist assigned to each patient a Kurtzke Disability Status Scale score and a Functional Systems Scale score.[22,23] We used the Incapacity Status Scale[24] to assess fatiguability. Thirty-six percent of the patients had relapsing-remitting MS, 50 percent had chronic progressive MS, and 14 percent were in transition between the two. The mean age of the patients at onset of MS symptoms was 29.1 years (s.d. 8.8) and the average length of illness was 11.3 years (s.d. 7.7), ranging from 1 to 34 years. Thirty-six percent of the patients were minimally disabled, 18 percent were moderately disabled, 30 percent required an aid to walk, and 16 percent required a wheelchair but could transfer independently. Twenty-nine patients (58%) were unable to carry out any sustained activity because of fatigue. The patients were similar to the large comparison sample except for more fatiguability ($\chi^2 = 10.57$, df = 3, $P = <0.05$). Five patients were in exacerbation and 12 were in hospital awaiting experimental treatment with ACTH and cyclophosphamide ($n = 11$) or plasmapheresis ($n = 1$).

Results

Rates of affective disorder

We determined lifetime rates for affective disorder in the MS group and compared them to rates reported in the literature for a community[25,26] and a medical population[27] using χ^2 contingency tests. Table 1 shows the lifetime prevalence rates for a number of disorders meeting the Research Diagnostic Criteria in the MS group and in the comparison populations, and whether the first psychiatric episode occurred prior to or following the onset of the MS. For major depression, minor depression, intermittent depression, hypomania, and any disorder meeting the Research Diagnostic Criteria, the MS patients had significantly more episodes. Similar comparisons of current and 1 year prevalence rates using DSM III (American Psychiatric Association, Diagnostic and Statistical Manual, third edition) criteria showed the same pattern.[28,29] Using proportionately age-weighted lifetime major depression rates for persons 26–45 and 46–55 years old, we found that the rate for major depression prior to MS (14%) was comparable to general population rates, but that the rate for major depression after the onset of MS (54%) was significantly greater (two-tailed comparisons of proportions, for the 26–45 year age group, $Z = 1.19$, $P > 0.10$ and for the 46–55 year age group, $Z = 4.60$, $P < 0.01$).[25]

All the hypomanic and manic episodes occurred during treatment with ACTH ($n = 8$) or prednisone ($n = 1$). There was one case each of alcoholism, phobic disorder, and schizo-affective disorder, all of which preceded the MS, and four cases of labile personality preceding the MS and one following it.

To determine whether the high rate of depression simply reflected the well known increase in depression among the medically ill or whether it was more specific to MS, we compared the mean Beck Depression Inventory scores of our patients with those of other medical patients reported in the literature, using two-tailed t-tests. Where means were not given, we took the

Table 1. *Lifetime rates of affective disorders according to the Research Diagnostic Criteria in MS patients and comparison populations*

Disorders	*Prior to MS (%)* ($n = 50$)	*Since MS (%)* ($n = 50$)	*Lifetime, MS (%)* ($n = 50$)	New Haven[25] 1975–76 (%) ($n = 511$)
Major depression	14	54	54	20[a]
Minor depression	8	52	52	9.2[a]
Intermittent depression	4	28	28	3.2[a,b]
Hypomania	2	14	16	0.8[a]
Mania	0	2	2	0.8
Generalized anxiety	4	12	16	—
Any disorder	36	84	84	49.5[c,d]

[a]χ^2 test (1 d.f.) *vs* lifetime MS rate: $P < 0.005$.
[b]New Haven, 1980–81,[26] $n = 3058$, DSM III diagnostic criteria.
[c]χ^2 test (1 d.f.) *vs* lifetime MS rate: $P < 0.05$.
[d]Primary Care patients,[27] $n = 247$, Research Diagnostic Criteria.

percentage of patients in the comparison study who were above the cut-off score used in that study and compared them with the percentage of our patients above that same cut-off score (Table 2). We used Fisher's Exact tests for small control populations and χ^2 tests for large control populations. The mean Beck score for the MS patients was 12.7 (s.d. 8.4) and 40 percent of the patients were above a cutting score of 14. Table 2 shows that the MS patients were more depressed than a group of general medical outpatients,[30] two groups of general medical inpatients,[31,32] and a group of cancer inpatients.[33] They were as depressed as a group of neurological outpatients,[1] another group of cancer inpatients,[34] and a group of general medical outpatients,[35] although the authors of the last two studies noted that their depression scores were likely to have been inflated because of some unusual characteristics of their patients.

Clinical features of depression

While 34 percent of patients met the criteria for major depression over the preceding year, many more were troubled by depression (64%), anger (64%), irritability (56%), worry (48%), discouragement (42%), and self-reproach (38%). Thirty-eight percent of patients were preoccupied with their bodies, 38 percent had difficulty concentrating, 36 percent had withdrawn from friends and family and another 36 percent thought poorly of themselves. Thirty-four percent described chronic anxiety and 28 percent had lost interest in their usual activities. While five patients had moderately serious suicidal preoccupations over the past year, none made a suicide attempt. Over the course of their illness, six patients made 10 suicide attempts; two were moderately serious.

We determined the subtypes of the major depressions suffered by the patients in the year prior to the study and compared these to a group of depressed outpatients[36] and a group comprised mainly of depressed inpatients[37] using Fisher's Exact tests. Ninety-six percent of the patients with major depression had had no previous psychiatric disorder other than depression (primary subtype), a rate similar to the outpatient comparison group, but significantly lower than the inpatient group ($P<0.05$). Sixty-seven percent of depressions were classified as recurrent unipolar depressions, indicating that patients had had two or more major depressive episodes. This rate was not significantly different from the rates for the comparison groups. Among the MS patients there were no psychotic, agitated, or retarded depressions and only two patients were so severely incapacitated by depression that they could not carry out their usual activities at work or at home. The MS patients had significantly fewer endogenous depressions than the inpatients (41% *vs* 87%, $P<0.01$), and more situational depressions than both comparison groups ($P<0.01$ for both comparisons). A situational depression is defined as one that 'developed after an event

Table 2. *Beck Depression Inventory scores in MS patients and comparison groups*

	n	*Mean (s.d.)*	*P*	*Percent above cut-off*	*P*
MS Patients	50	12.7(8.4)		40[c]	
Comparison Group					
General medical outpatients[30]	526	5.9(5.4)	<0.01	12.2[b]	<0.005
General medical inpatients[31]	153	9.7(6.6)	<0.03	22[c]	<0.02
General medical inpatients[32]	120	—	—	24[c]	<0.05
Cancer inpatients[33]	97	9.6	<0.05	23[c]	<0.04
Neurological outpatients[1]	30	—	—	26.7[d]	>0.05
Cancer inpatients[34]	62	—	—	33[c]	>0.05
Medical outpatients[35]	80	11.2(7.5)	—	48[a]	>0.05

Cut-off scores: [a] $\geqslant 11$ [b] $\geqslant 13$ [c] $\geqslant 14$ [d] $\geqslant 15$

or in a situation that seems likely to have contributed to the appearance of the episode at that time.'[17] The MS patients had more simple depressions than the outpatients ($P<0.05$), meaning that they showed 'no significant signs of psychiatric disturbance in the year prior to the development of the current' depression except for symptoms of depression or mania.[17]

Predictors of depression

A major purpose of this study was to see if we could predict who would have a major depression. Using the major depressions in the year preceding the study, since the patients' recall about these was most accurate, we compared the 17 patients who had had major depressions with the 33 who had not in terms of a number of possible risk factors, using Fisher's Exact tests applied to two-by-two contingency tables. The occurrence of a major depression was related to a history of major depression prior to the onset of MS symptoms ($P<0.01$) and a history of major depression since the onset of MS symptoms ($P<0.01$). The depressions were more likely to have been preceded within a month by an MS exacerbation that was treated with ACTH or prednisone ($P<0.01$). Preceding major life events such as loss of a job or severe marital discord did not distinguish the patients with major depressions from the others (Fisher's Exact test, $P>0.05$), nor did severity of disability, duration of symptoms, age, socioeconomic status (Mann-Whitney tests, $P>0.05$ for all comparisons), type of MS or gender (χ^2 tests, $P>0.05$ for the last two variables).

The severity of depressive symptoms as measured by the Beck Depression Inventory was unrelated to the severity of disability, functional system involvement, duration of MS, fatiguability, age, socioeconomic status (Pearson product-moment correlations, $P>0.05$ for all comparisons), type of MS, current clinical status (exacerbation *vs* remission) and gender (Mann-Whitney tests, $P>0.05$ for all comparisons).

Family history of depression

We also wanted to see if family history of affective disorder influenced the overall rate of major depression. Using Fisher's Exact tests we compared the rate of major depression developing after the onset of MS in patients with a family history of unipolar depression and alcoholism (either depression or alcoholism or both) to the rate of major depression in patients with no family psychiatric history at all. We performed similar analyses looking at the rate of major depression developing before the onset of MS.

Neither the rate of major depression since the onset of MS nor the rate of major depression prior to the onset of MS was different in patients with family histories of unipolar depression or alcoholism or depression and/or alcoholism as compared to patients with no family psychiatric history at all. Of the 27 patients whose first major depression followed their MS, 11 had family histories of depression and/or alchololism while of the 23 patients who had no major depression following their MS, six had family histories of depression and/or alcoholism ($P=0.44$). Of the seven patients whose first major depression preceded their MS, four had family histories of depression and/or alcoholism, while of the 43 patients who did not have a major depression prior to their MS, 14 had family histories of depression and/or alcoholism ($P=0.44$).

Psychiatric Treatment

Only 24 of the 40 patients who met Research Diagnostic Criteria for any psychiatric disorder over the preceding year underwent some sort of psychiatric treatment: 10 received lithium or tricyclic antidepressants, nine took minor tranquilizers intermittently, two received major tranquilizers, three saw a mental health professional for one visit and 15 had at least 2 weeks of psychotherapy. One patient was hospitalized for psychiatric reasons. Twenty-five patients had no psychiatric treatment of any kind.

Discussion

Among these 50 moderately disabled MS patients there were high rates of all depressive disorders. These rates had increased significantly from the period before MS symptoms began. Fifty-four percent of the patients had had at least one major depression since the onset of their MS symptoms. At the time of the study the MS patients were more depressed than other groups of medical patients and even those who did not meet the full criteria for major depression complained of depressive symptoms. The depressions were mild to moderately severe and characterized by symptoms of dysphoria, anger, irritability, worry, and discouragement rather than by self-criticism, withdrawal, loss of interest, and suicidal preoccupation.

We were able to isolate two clinical predictors of major depression: first, a past history of major depression beginning either before or after the onset of the illness; second, a preceding exacerbation of the MS that was treated with ACTH or prednisone. Unfortunately we had too few patients who either received these medications when stable or who were not treated during an exacerbation to determine whether disease activity, medication, of the combination of the two was the key factor. The depressions were not associated with the severity of disability, a particular functional system, duration of illness, type of MS, clinical status, fatiguability, age, sex or socioeconomic status. In addition, the patients with major depressions were not distinguished from the others by family histories of depression or alcoholism.

Can these results shed light on the possible mechanisms of association between MS and depression? The findings in this study, particularly the comparisons with other medical populations and the relationship between depression and treated exacerbation, suggest that MS itself directly contributes to the occurrence of depression. While the absence of positive family histories in the depressed patients suggests that these patients did not have a primary affective disorder, the greater frequency of depression prior to MS suggests the opposite. Nevertheless, it would be a misuse of clinical data to presume an etiology for the depressive episodes and it is most likely that the depressions result from a complex interaction of a number of variables, including the pathophysiology of the disease, the particular stresses imposed by the disease, and the genetic, psychological, and social characteristics of individual patients. It is not surprising that major depressions were often preceded by exacerbations treated with ACTH or prednisone. In addition to the potential for these medications to produce psychiatric reactions,[38,39] the demyelinating process and such psychological factors as grief, fear, and discouragement will have their strongest effect when the disease is active. It is similarly not surprising that the severity of disability as measured by the Disability Status Scale was unrelated to depression. Unlike the sudden deterioration that occurs during an exacerbation, the degree of disability a patient experiences generally has evolved gradually over the course of the illness and has allowed time for emotional and social adjustment.

The findings of this study are limited by the relatively small sample size, and by the fact that patients came from a specialized teaching hospital and that much of the data on depressive disorders were retrospective. Actual comparisons to other medical patients matched for age and type of disability would be preferable to using literature samples. The considerable variability among the patients in characteristics such as disability may obscure subtle but meaningful relationships.

The clinical implications of our findings are important. The low rate of treatment for depression is a matter for concern and the high rate of chronic intermittent depression[40] indicates either that current treatment practices are not adequate or that the depressions are peculiarly resistant to standard treatments. Clinicians need to be more aggressive in detecting and treating depression and patients and family members should be made aware of the risk of depression and encouraged to seek treatment when indicated. Patients at risk, that is, those with past histories of depression and those being treated for an exacerbation, should be alerted to the possibility of becoming depressed and watched for symptoms. The high degree of depressive symptomatology in patients who did not meet formal criteria for major depression suggests that there is a spectrum of depressive disorders, including normal grief and discouragement, adjustment reaction with depressed mood, and dysthymic disorder. Treatment should be tailored to the individual patient and may include individual psychotherapy, couple and family therapy, and medication.

Acknowledgements. The study was supported in part by NIMH grant MH15531, the Ethel Dupont-Warren Fellowship, the Bretholtz Multiple Sclerosis Fund, the Peter B. Livingston Fellowship Fund, the Milton Fund, NIH Grant RR05489 awarded to the Brigham and Women's Hospital, and the G. Gorham Peters Trust.

The authors thank Drs H. Richard Tyler, David M. Dawson, Howard L. Weiner, David A. Hafler, and Stephen Hauser for their neurological evaluations of the subjects.

The data in this paper were originally published as 'Depression in Multiple Sclerosis' in *General Hospital Psychiatry* **9**, 426-434, 1987, and the paper is reprinted with minor changes by permission of Elsevier Science Publishing Co. Inc.

References

1 Whitlock, F. A. & Siskind M. M. (1980): Depression as a major symptom of multiple sclerosis. *J. Neurol. Neurosurg. Psychiatry* **48**, 361–365.

2 Surridge, D. (1969): An investigation into some psychiatric aspects of multiple sclerosis. *Br. J. Psychiatry* **115**, 749–764.

3 Schiffer, R. B., Caine E. D., Bamford K. A., *et al.* (1988): Depressive episodes in patients with multiple sclerosis. *Am. J. Psychiatry* **140**, 1498–1500.

4 Pratt, R. T. C. (1951): An investigation of the psychiatric aspects of disseminated sclerosis. *J. Neurol. Neurosurg. Psychiatry* **14**, 326–335.

5 Dalos, N. P., Rabins, P. V., Brooks, B. R., *et al.* (1983): Disease activity and emotional state in multiple sclerosis. *Ann. Neurol.* **13**, 573–583.

6 Cleeland, C. S., Matthews C. G. & Hopper, C. L. (1970): MMPI profiles in exacerbation and remission of multiple sclerosis. *Psychol. Rep.* **27**, 373–374.

7 Rabins, P. V., Brooks, B. R., O'Donnell, P., *et al.* (1986): Structural brain correlates of emotional disorder in multiple sclerosis. *Brain* **109**, 585–597.

8 McIvor, G. P., Riklan, M. & Reznikoff, M. (1984): Depression in multiple sclerosis as a function of length and severity of illness, age, remissions, and perceived social support. *J. Clin. Psychol.* **40**, 1028–1033.

9 Jambor, K. L. (1969): Cognitive functioning in multiple sclerosis. *Br. J. Psychiatry* **115**, 765–775.

10 Peyser, J. M., Edwards, K. R., Poser, C. M., *et al.* (1980): Cognitive function in patients with multiple sclerosis. *Arch. Neurol.* **37**, 577–579.

11 Rao, S. M., Hammeke, T. A., McQuillen, M. P., *et al.* (1984): Memory disturbance in chronic progressive multiple sclerosis. *Arch. Neurol.* **41**, 625–631.

12 Vowels, L. M. & Gates, G. R. (1984): Neuropsychological findings. In *Multiple sclerosis: Psychological and social aspects*, ed A. F. Simons, pp 82–90. London: Heinemann.

13 Schumacher, G. A., Beebe G., Kibler, R. F., *et al.* (1965): Problems of experimental trials of therapy in multiple sclerosis: report by the panel on the evaluation of experimental trials of therapy in multiple sclerosis. *Ann. N.Y. Acad. Sci.* **122**, 552–563.

14 Hollingshead, A. G.: Four-factor index of social status. A working paper. New Haven: Yale University.

15 LaRocca N. G., Scheinberg, L., Slater, R. J., *et al.* (1934): Field testing of a minimal record of disability in multiple sclerosis: The United States and Canada. *Acta Neurol. Scand.* **70**, 126–138.
16 Endicott, J. & Spitzer, R. L. (1978): A diagnostic interview: The schedule for affective disorders and schizophrenia. *Arch. Gen. Psychiatry* **35**, 837–844.
17 Spitzer, R. L., Endicott, J. & Robins, E. (1978): Research diagnostic criteria: Rationale and reliability. *Arch. Gen. Psychiatry* **35**, 773–782.
18 Endicott, J. & Spitzer, R. L. (1979): Use of the research diagnostic criteria and the schedule for affective disorders and schizophrenia to study affective disorders. *Am. J. Psychiatry* **136**, 52–56.
19 Endicott, J., Andreasen, N. & Spitzer, R. L. (1975) : *Family History—Research Diagnostic Criteria.* New York: Biometrics Research, New York State Psychiatric Institute.
20 Andreasen, N. C, Endicott, J., Spitzer, R. L., *et al.* (1977): Family history method using diagnostic criteria. *Arch. Gen. Psychiatry* **34**, 1229–1235.
21 Beck, A. T., Ward, C. H., Mendelson, M., *et al.* (1961): An inventory for measuring depression. *Arch. Gen. Psychiatry* **4**: 561–571.
22 Kurtzke, J. F. (1961): On the evaluation of disability in multiple sclerosis. *Neurology* **11**, 686–694.
23 Kurtzke, J. F. (1965): Further notes on disability evaluation in multiple sclerosis with scale modifications. *Neurology* **15**, 654–661.
24 International Federation of Multiple Sclerosis Societies (1984): *Minimal record of disability for multiple sclerosis.* New York: National Multiple Sclerosis Society.
25 Weissman, M. M. & Myers, J. K. (1978): Affective disorders in a U.S. urban community. The use of research diagnostic criteria in an epidemiological survey. *Arch. Gen. Psychiatry* **35**, 1304–1311.
26 Robins, L. N., Helzer, J. E., Weissman, M. M., *et al.* (1984): Lifetime prevalence of specific psychiatric disorders in three sites. *Arch. Gen. Psychiatry* **41**, 949–958.
27 Hoeper, E. W., Nycz, G. R., Cleary, P. D., *et al.* (1979): Estimated prevalence of RDC mental disorder in primary medical care. *Int. J. Ment. Health* **8**, 6–15.
28 Roberts, R. E. & Vernon, S. W. (1982): Depression in the community: Prevalence and treatment. *Arch. Gen. Psychiatry* **39**, 1407–1409.
29 Myers, J. K., Weissman, M. M., Tischler, G. L., *et al.* (1984): Six-month prevalence of psychiatric disorders in three communities. *Arch. Gen. Psychiatry* **41**, 959–967.
30 Nielsen III A. C. & Williams, T. A. (1980): Depression in ambulatory medical patients. *Arch. Gen. Psychiatry* **37**, 999–1004.
31 Schwab, J., Bialow, M., Clemmons, R., *et al.* (1967): The Beck Depression Inventory with medical inpatients. *Acta Psychiatr. Scand.* **43**, 255–266.
32 Moffic, H. & Paykel, E. S. (1975): Depression in medical in-patients. *Br. J. Psychiatry* **126**, 346–353.
33 Plumb, M. M. & Holland, J. (1977): Comparative studies of psychological function in patients with advanced cancer—1. Self-reported depressive symptoms. *Psychosom. Med.* **39**, 264–276.
34 Bukberg, J., Penman, D. & Holland, J. C. (1984): Depression in hospitalized cancer patients. *Psychom. Med.* **46**, 199–212.
35 Salkind, M. R. (1969): Beck depression inventory in general practice. *J. R. Coll. Gen. Pract.* **18**, 267–273.
36 Prusoff, B. A., Weissman, M. M., Klerman, G. L., *et al.* (1980): Research diagnostic criteria subtypes of depression. *Arch. Gen. Psychiatry* **37**, 796–801.
37 Keller, M. B., Klerman, G. L., Lavori, P. W., *et al.* (1982): Treatment received by depressed patients. *JAMA* **248**, 1848–1855.
38 Ling, M. H. M., Perry, P. J. & Tsuang, M. T. (1981): Side effects of corticosteroid therapy. *Arch. Gen. Psychiatry* **38**, 471–477.
39 Lewis, D. A. & Smith, R. E. (1983): Steroid-induced psychiatric syndromes. A report of 14 cases and a review of the literature. *J. Affective Disord.* **5**, 319–332.
40 Weissman, M. M. & Klerman, G. L. (1977): The chronic depressive in the community: Unrecognized and poorly treated. *Compr. Psychiatry* **18**, 523–532.

VI

MENTAL DISORDERS AND COGNITION

15

COGNITIVE IMPAIRMENT, EMOTIONAL DISTURBANCES AND DURATION OF MULTIPLE SCLEROSIS

R. Jouvent*, M. Montreuil*†, N. Benoit†. C. Lubetzki†, E. Tournier-Lasserve†, A. des Lauriers*, D. Widlocher*, F. Lhermitte†, O. Lyon-Caen†

**INSERM U 302 Psychopathologie et Psychopharmacologie des comportements La Salpêtrière, 47 Bd de l'hôpital, 75013 Paris; and*
†Clinique de Neurologie et de Neuropsychologie La Salpêtrière, Paris, France

Summary

A collaborative study between neurologists, psychiatrists and psychologists was organized at the Salpêtrière Hospital in Paris, in order to evaluate the influence of the duration of multiple sclerosis (MS) on cognitive and affective impairment. Two groups of patients, one with MS or recent optic neuritis of less than 2 years duration, the second one with more than 6 and less than 12 years duration, were compared. Results showed a cognitive impairment in 46 percent of early MS patients *vs* 68 percent in the long-standing group. There was a significantly greater likelihood of depression in the recent onset group (38% *vs* 17%). Depression and cognitive impairment were not correlated. However there was a strong link between affective incontinence and cognitive impairment. Theoretical and methodological issues are discussed.

Introduction

Mental, cognitive and mood disorders in multiple sclerosis (MS) have been well known phenomena ever since Charcot's (1868) and Vulpian's (1874) original reports. However, their incidence, occurrence and natural history are not precisely defined. This is probably due in part to the heterogeneity of the groups of patients studied. Depression has been described with varying frequency in MS.[1,2] These conflicting reports about the prevalence of depression may reflect inter-study differences in patient selection and in the criteria used for the diagnosis of depression. Another major problem accounting for differences in the estimates of concomitant depression in MS patients is the similarity of signs and symptoms in both illnesses. This overlap of symptoms may account for both elevated depression scores and depressed cognitive scores. On the other hand, the influence of depression upon cognitive disturbances in MS has not been well studied. To clear up these two main points, a collaborative study between neurologists, psychiatrists and psychologists was organized at the Salpêtrière Hospital in Paris.

Methods

In order to evaluate the influence of the duration of MS, we compared two groups of patients: the first consisted of 37 patients (age 29.5 years, s.d. 5.9) with MS or recent optic neuritis of less than 2 years' duration. The second group consisted of 35 patients (age 36.6 years, s.d. 9.8) with MS for more than 6 and less than 12 years' duration. MS was classified as probable or definite according to the criteria of Poser *et al.*.[3] The patients were classified according to their cultural level (CL) (CL 1 = school learning for a trade; CL 2 = 2–6 years' secondary schooling after 14; CL 3 = more than 6 years of secondary schooling). All of these patients had a normal social life and none of them complained of memory disturbance. Results of these two groups were compared to those of a control group of 27 patients.

Neuropsychological evaluation

Testing protocol was designed to be simple and standardized, with results adjusted to the CL.[4] Because of a possible functional handicap, tests using spoken vocabulary, visuo-spatial interpretation and drawing were excluded.

Intellectual efficiency was studied with the Wechsler Adult Intelligence Scale (WAIS) and the Wisconsin Card Sorting Test (WCST). Three subtests of WAIS were selected: vocabulary, similarities and cubes. The procedure utilized for the Wisconsin Test was that described by Nelson.[5] Memory performances were assessed by the complete Wechsler Memory Scale.

Impairment was considered definite if two or three subtests of WAIS and/or two or three subtests of Wechsler Memory Scale and mnestic quotient were below the normal lower level. If only one of these tests was abnormal, two situations were possible: (1) the total score was superior or equal to the lower theoretical level, in which case the patient was considered normal; (2) the total was under the lower theoretical level, in which case the patient was considered to have a probable impairment (doubtful result).

Psychiatric evaluation

On the same day, patients were independently rated by a research psychologist. The evaluation comprised DSM III criteria for a major depressive episode,[6] Echelle de Ralentissement Depressif[8] (ERD), Hamilton Depression Rating scale,[9] Echelle d'Humeur Depressive[10] (EHD).

Results and discussion

We present here preliminary analysis of this collaborative programme.

Neuropsychological data

In cases of early MS and recently isolated optic neuritis, 46 percent of patients had cognitive impairment and 11 percent had doubtful results. Abnormalities were always mild to moderate. Verbal and non-verbal efficiencies were simultaneously disturbed in nearly all the cases. Memory difficulties were present both visually and verbally. In all these cases, tests for calculation, naming construction and verbal fluency were normal. No perseveration, slowness in execution or indifference were observed. Comparison with the control group showed significant differences for all the tests except two (cube for CL 3; span for CL 2).

Long-standing MS (between 6 and 12 years' duration), 68 percent of patients had cognitive impairment. Abnormalities observed in this population were heterogeneous. Disorientation and confabulation were never observed.

Cognitive impairment in MS is frequent even in patients who do not complain of any symptoms and lead a normal life. It may easily escape detection if not specifically looked for.[11,12] The impairment may be dissociated, that is, memory and intellectual performances can be impaired separately. Learning abilities are preserved in MS of recent onset.

There was no relationship between cognitive impairment and the degree of handicap or the clinical course of the disease. These results are in line with those of Rao *et al.*[13] and contrast with data of Grant *et al.*[11]

Cognitive impairment probably increases with the progression of MS but its frequency is not significantly different.

In the cases in which nuclear magnetic resonance (NMR) imaging was performed, cognitive impairment was always associated with NMR signal abnormalities.

Multifactorial analysis of neuropsychological tests

Principal components analysis of the cognitive variables was performed for the whole population. The results are summarized in Table 1, which shows correlations between the variables and two factors after Varimax rotation. The factors are a general cognitive factor (factor 1) which included all the tests, and an individualized factor (factor 2) which primarily included the Wisconsin Card Sorting Test. Factor 1 accounted for more than 58% of the variance and factor 2 for 11%.

Figure 1 shows a graphic projection of factor scores of the two groups of patients. Although there were global similarities between the two populations, there were also some

Table 1. *Orthogonal transformation solution—Varimax.*

	Factor 1	*Factor 2*
WAIS cubes	0.773	−0.056
WAIS similarities	0.799	0.388
WAIS vocabulary	0.796	0.179
WMS mnesic quotient	0.932	−0.208
WMS story	0.786	−0.179
WMS pattern	0.762	−0.288
Digit Span	0.579	−0.407
WCST	0.62	0.614

WAIS = Wechsler Adult Intelligence Scale; WMS = Wechsler Memory Scale; WCST = Wisconsin Card Sorting Test.

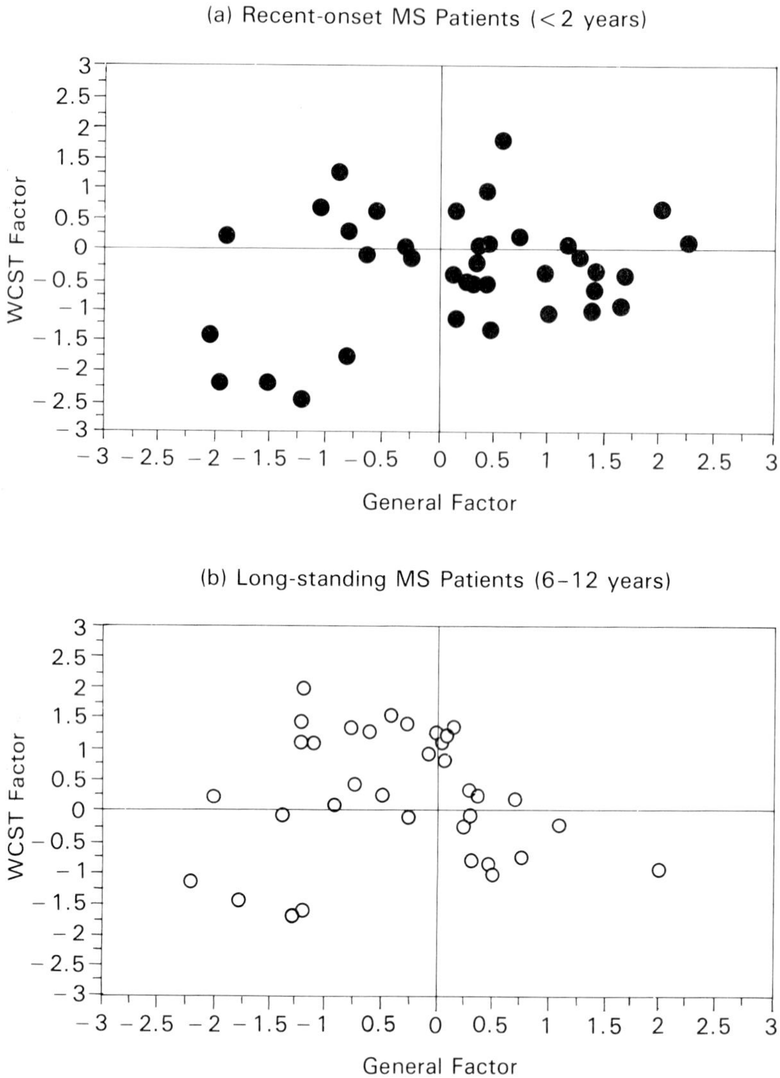

Fig. 1. *Projection of patients on two axes of factor analysis.* In long-standing MS, very few patients have a combined high general factor and low WCST (Wisconsin Card Sorting Test), which may be interpreted as a depressive pattern.

specific differences. Thus fewer patients in the recent onset (<2 years) group had low scores on factor 1, while the long duration (6–12 years) group were more likely to have low factor 1 and high factor 2 scores.

Course of cognitive disorders

In the recent onset group we were able to re-examine 25 patients 12 to 18 months after the first examination. In the eight cases where a global cognitive impairment was observed, this was still present one year later. Among 10 patients with normal cognitive function at the first examination, nine were still normal 12 months later, and one had doubtful results. Of seven patients with doubtful results at the first examination, two were normal and one was definitely abnormal 1 year later.

Psychopathological data

Depression. The comparison between recent onset and long-standing MS in relation to DSM III criteria for major depressive illness shows a significant difference between the groups. In the recent onset group, 14 out of 37 patients (38%) fulfilled depression criteria, whereas in the long duration group, only six out of 35 (17%) fulfilled the criteria (χ^2-test: $P = 0.05$). The recent onset group also had a significantly higher Hamilton Depression Rating Scale score (14.9, s.d. 1.1, *vs* 11.7, s.d. 1.2, t-test $P < 0.04$).

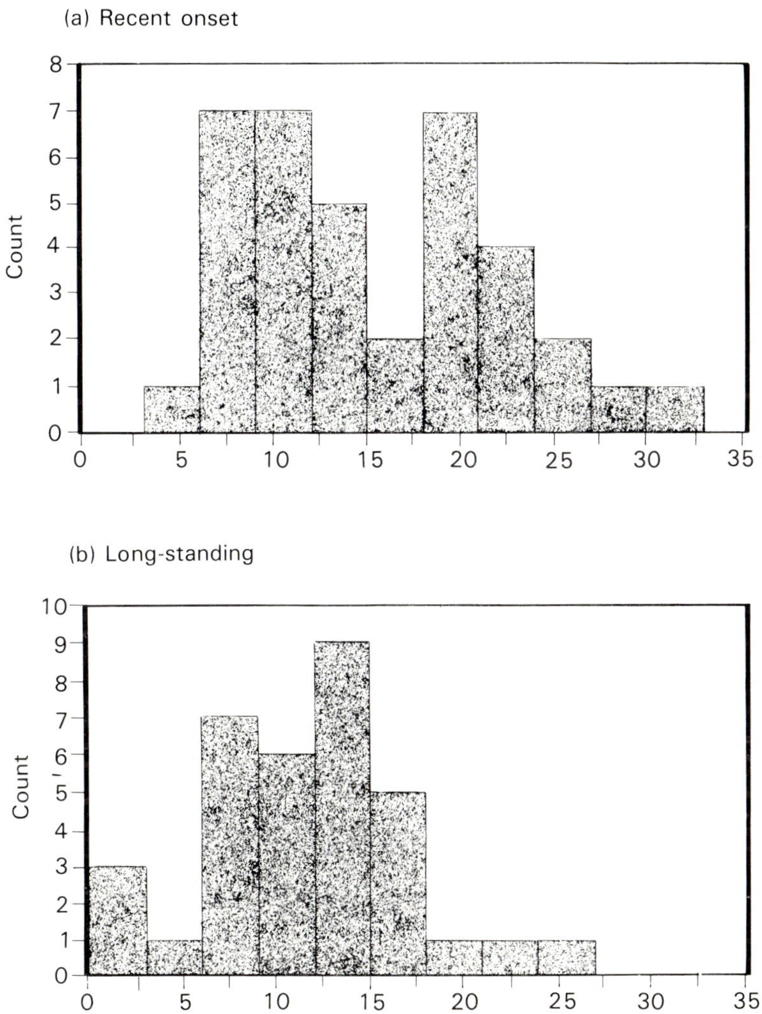

Fig. 2. *Comparison of Hamilton Depression Rating scores in MS patients with disease of recent onset and long-standing disease.*

Nevertheless Fig. 2 shows that these differences comprise a bimodal *versus* a unimodal distribution. In the population with long-standing disease very few patients were depressed and the distribution was unimodal, whereas the recent onset population could be divided into euthymic and depressed subgroups.

Interaction between affective variables and cognitive impairments

We did not find a correlation between degree of cognitive impairment and depressive symptoms but the depressed patients nevertheless had more cognitive impairment, in line with Jambor's findings.[14] In particular, some affective symptoms appeared to be correlated with cognitive variables. In the recent onset group, affective incontinence (as measured by EHD[10]) correlated with mnesic quotient, stories, cubes and the general cognitive factor (factor 1). In the group with long-standing disease, this item correlated only with similitudes. This is an argument in favour of a link between cognitive impairment and emotional incontinence, in spite of the absence of cognitive specificity for this symptom. These results are in line with previous findings by our group.[15]

Theoretical considerations

One of the major problems in psychiatric research concerns the heterogeneity of patients. Table 2 shows the cases of two patients both meeting DSM III criteria for a major depressive episode. They differed in various ways, so we had difficulty comparing them from the neuropsychological as well as from the psychopathological point of view. For example a cognitive test of attention is evidently different when patients have insomnia or hypersomnia. Criteriology is useful in comparing two global treatments or in epidemiology. It is not so adequate for correlation studies between clinical and neuropsychological variables.

It might be hypothesized that some neuropsychological and psychopathological signs are relatively simple whereas others are derived from a complex synthesis of different

Table 2. *DSM III criteria for major depressive episode.*

(A) Dysphoric mood or loss of interest or pleasure

(B) At least four of the following symptoms have each been present nearly every day for a period of at least 2 weeks:

(1) Poor appetite or significant weight loss or increased appetite or significant weight gain.
(2) Insomnia or hypersomnia.
(3) Psychomotor agitation or retardation.
(4) Loss of interest or pleasure in usual activities, or decrease in sexual drive.
(5) Loss of energy; fatigue.
(6) Feelings of worthlessness, self-reproach, or excessive or inappropriate guilt.
(7) Complaints or evidence of diminished ability to think or concentrate, such as slowed thinking, or indecisiveness not associated with marked loosening of associations or incoherence.
(8) Recurrent thoughts of death, suicidal ideas, wishes to be dead, or suicide attempt.

Patient A had:	*Patient B had:*
—psychomotor agitation	—retardation
—insomnia	—hypersomnia
—increased appetite	—fatigue
—excessive guilt	—loss of interest

elements coming from various levels of observation. In depressed patients we showed a splitting up of depressive mood into several different dimensions. Indeed five clinically and statistically coherent factors may be isolated from EHD: blunted affect, hyperexpressive sadness/affective incontinence, irritability, affective lability, and visible signs of mental suffering.[16] This provides evidence that depressive mood is a general concept and not a clinical entity. Some dimensions, such as affective lability or incontinence, are relatively simple, and thus may be correlated to neuropsychological performance. Some others are more complex. The comparison between cognitive and affective variables in MS should examine these considerations.

References

1 Surridge, D. (1969): An investigation into some psychiatric aspects of multiple sclerosis. *Br. J. Psychiatry* **115**, 479–764.

2 Whitlock, F. A. & Siskind, M. M. (1980): Depression as a major symptom of multiple sclerosis. *J. Neurol. Neurosurg. Psychiatry* **43**, 861.

3 Poser, C. M., Paty, D. W., Scheinberg, L. *et al.* (1983): New diagnostic criteria for multiple sclerosis: guidelines for research protocols. *Ann. Neurol.* **13**, 227–231.

4 Perse, J. (1972): Collaboration du psychologue au dépistage et au diagnostic des maladies mentales. In *Traité de psychologie appliquée* vol 8. ed M. Reuchlin, pp 109–147. Paris: Presses Universitaires de France.

5 Nelson, H. E. (1976): A modified card sorting test sensitive to frontal lobe defects. *Cortex* **12**, 313–324.

6 *Diagnostic and statistical manual of mental disorders* (1980). 3rd ed. Washington: American Psychiatric Association.

7 Poitrenaud, J., Barrere, H. & Moreau, C. (1973): Influence de l'âge sur quelques unes des principales dimensions non cognitives de la personnalité. *Gerontologia* **19**, 31–44

8 Widlöcher, D., ed (1983): *Le ralentissement dépressif*, pp 7–25. Paris: Presses Universitaires de France.

9 Hamilton, M. (1967): Development of a rating scale for primary depressive illness. *Br. J. Soc. Clin. Psychol.* **6**, 278–296.

10 Jouvent, R., Hardy, P., Bouvard, M., Braconnier, A., Roumengous, V., Grasset, F. & Widlöcher, D. (1987): L'hétérogénéité de l'humeur dépressive: Construction d'une échelle polydimentionnelle. *Encéphale* **13**, 233–237.

11 Grant, I., McDonald, W. I., Trimble, M. R. *et al.* (1984): Deficient learning and memory in early and middle phases of multiple sclerosis. *J. Neurol. Neurosurg. Psychiatry* **47**, 250–255.

12 Peyser, J. M., Edwards, K. R., Poser, C. M. *et al.* (1980): Cognitive function in patients with multiple sclerosis. *Arch. Neurol.* **37**, 577–579.

13 Rao, S. M., Glatt, S., Hammeke, T. A. *et al.* (1985): Chronic progressive multiple sclerosis: relationship between cerebral ventricular size and neuropsychological impairment. *Arch. Neurol.* **42**, 678–682.

14 Jambor, K. L. (1969): Cognitive functioning in MS. *Br. J. Psychiatry* **115**, 765–775.

15 Lyon-Caen, O., Jouvent, R., Hauser, S., Chaunu, M. P., Benoit, N., Widlöcher, D. & Lhermitte, F. (1986): Cognitive functions in recent multiple sclerosis and optic neuritis. *Arch. Neurol.* **43**, 1138–1148.

16 Jouvent, R., Vindreau, C., Montreuil, M., Bungener, C. & Widlöcher, D. (1988): La clinique polydimensionnelle de l'humeur dépressive. Nouvelle version de l'échelle EHD. *Psychiatr. Psychobiol.* **3**, 245–253.

16

CORRELATION OF BECK DEPRESSION INVENTORY SCORE, KURTZKE DISABILITY STATUS SCALE AND COGNITIVE FUNCTIONING IN MULTIPLE SCLEROSIS

Egon Stenager, Lone Knudsen, and Knud Jensen

Clinical Neuropsychiatric Research Unit, Departments of Neurology, Clinical Psychology and Psychiatry, Odense University Hospital, Odense, Denmark

Summary

A representative group of 114 patients with definite multiple sclerosis (MS) have completed the Beck Depression Inventory. Patients with Kurtzke Disability Status Scale grades 4–6 had significantly higher depression scores than the rest of the patients. Patients with evident decline in cognitive function had the highest depression scores indicating that the association between MS and affective diseases is due to cognitive dysfunction in MS patients.

Introduction

The subject of this chapter is the correlation between depressive symptoms, degree of physical disablement and cognitive function in patients with multiple sclerosis (MS). Many impressive investigations are described in the literature and they clearly show that depressive symptoms are frequently present in the MS patient—and are also believed to be associated with the disease.[1-6] It has been shown in several investigations that there is a correlation between the severity of the disease and depression,[7] in that the depression becomes more obvious with exacerbation of the disease[8] and progression in physical disablement,[9] although some have been unable to demonstrate this correlation.[10]

Only a few investigations have sought to correlate combined variables of depressive symptoms, degree of physical disability and cognitive function. Jambor[11] and Surridge[12] were the first to combine these variables. They used the same patients but published their work individually. Surridge believed that the depressive signs were a reactive condition, while Jambor remarked that 'patients suffering from multiple sclerosis tend to get symptoms of anxiety and depression in the initial stage of their lower intellectual efficiency'.

In a new investigation, Lyon-Caen *et al.*[13] concluded that 'there was no correlation with a depressive status between the presence of cognitive impairment and either the degree of handicap or the activity of the disease', while Rao *et al.*[14] found 'a group, showing mild memory disturbances, associated with the use of psychotropic medications and reactive depression'.

There are obviously conflicting opinions on the question of a correlation.

Material and methods

Our investigation covers 115 patients between 25 and 55 years of age with definite MS. They are selected so as to form a group that is representative of patients who were hospital inpatients in the neurological department, Odense University Hospital, in the period 1.4.1973–31.12.1985. They comprised 48 per cent of the patients in this age group suspected of having definite MS who lived in the geographical region of Funen. None of the patients had any current condition affecting the CNS of either primary or secondary nature, neither did they have alcoholism or any other chronic disease.

Permission to contact the patient was received from the general practitioner. The patients received a letter describing the investigation and its purpose. If the patient agreed to take part in the investigation he was visited at home, first by a physician and then within the succeeding 2–4 weeks by a neuropsychologist. These two researchers examined all the patients in question.

The physician collected anamnestic information, carried out a neurological examination and gave the patient a questionnaire to complete. Help for its completion was given to those whose motor deficits hindered them from writing. The neuropsychologist recorded the neuropsychological history of each patient and carried out the neuropsychological tests. Prior to her examination the medical findings were unknown to her, but she was aware of social problems and complaints of cognitive disturbance. Each visit lasted on average 3 hours.

The procedure was as follows: (1) Neurological examination was carried out and the patient's physical impairment was classified according to the Kurtzke Disability Status Scale (KDSS).[15] (2) The Beck Depression Inventory (BDI),[16] in a Danish version, was completed by the patient. (3) Neuropsychological examination was carried out.

The patients were divided into KDSS groups but some groups were combined to form larger ones. This was felt justified since the borderlines may be unclear in some cases.

Results

Of the 115 patients, only one was unwilling to complete the Beck Depression Inventory. Our study therefore included 114 patients.

The mean values of the BDI scores were calculated for each KDSS group. The resulting curve is shown in Fig. 1. The mean depression score increased with increasing KDSS up to and including KDSS 5–6. Non-parametric comparison of BDI scores for the groups shows that KDSS 4 and 5–6 diverged significantly from KDSS 1–2 and 3 ($P<0.02$). However, the tendency for depression to increase with worsening disability was not seen in those patients with the highest disability rating (KDSS 7–9) who had somewhat lower depression scores, equivalent to KDSS group 3. The mean BDI score for these patients did not differ significantly from the scores in the other groups. How can these findings be explained? To find an explanation, we must return to the curves for cognitive function in MS patients seen in Chapter 4. In Fig. 1 in that chapter (p 31) we saw that the patients with marked disability (KDSS 7–9) performed significantly worse than the others in the WAIS–R test of cognitive function and thus had evidence of severe brain damage. These

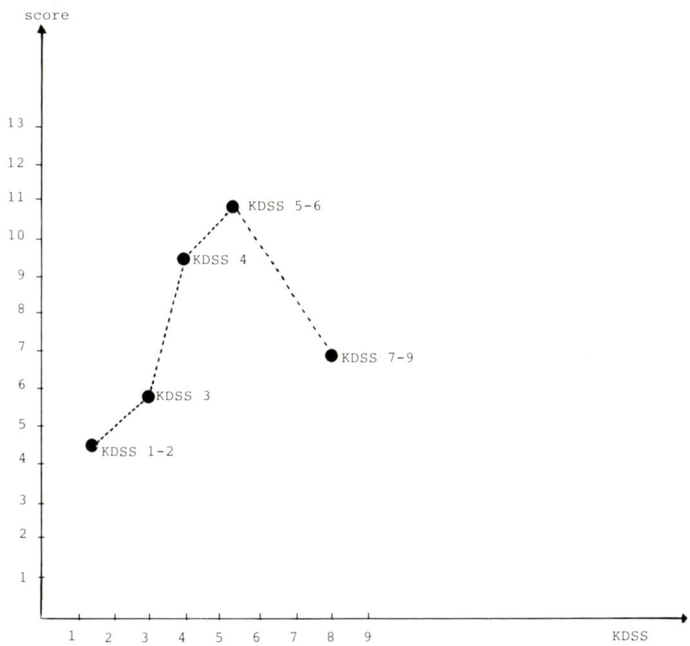

Figure. *Beck Depression Inventory* (BDI) versus *Kurtzke Disability Status Scale (KDSS)*. KDSS 1–2, $n=21$; 3, $n=36$; 4, $n=23$; 5–6, $n=19$; 7–9, $n=15$.

are the patients whose depression scores we have now shown to be less severe than in patients with milder degrees of disability. It appears therefore that those patients who are developing brain damage have more depression than those in whom brain damage has become severe. Similarly, in the Auditive Verbal Learning Test (Chapter 4, Fig. 2, p 32) the patients in the KDSS 7–9 group learned only a few words, which were quickly forgotten. These patients were less depressed than those in KDSS groups 4 and 5–6, with intermediate physical difficulty, who had obvious learning problems with reduced delayed recall but who were not yet seriously demented. The same pattern is repeated in the other cognitive tests described in Chapter 4 (Story Recall, Recurring Figures Test, Visual Gestalt Test, Trail Making and Symbol Digit Modalities). In all these tests, the patients with the most physical disability performed worst but were not especially depressed, while those with intermediate degrees of disability also performed poorly (though not so poorly as the KDSS 7–9 group) but were particularly depressed; in other words it was in the patients in whom intellectual deterioration was gaining speed that depression was most marked.

Discussion and Conclusions

We have found that the patients in the KDSS 7–9 group are intellectually severely damaged, as evaluated by the intelligence tests, and they particularly reveal damage of long-term memory evaluated on 'Information' and 'Vocabulary', and on all memory tests and attention and motor perceptual speed tests. We have then a picture of these patients that shows they have severe brain damage but no longer complain particularly of depressive symptoms, as shown by the BDI scores.

Patients in disability groups KDSS 4 and KDSS 5–6 present signs of decline in the intelligence tests. There is a distinct decline in both the verbal and visual memory and in attention and motor perceptual speed. It was these patients whose scores for depression were significantly higher in comparison with patients in KDSS 1–2 and KDSS 3 groups.

Compared with controls the patients in KDSS 1–2 groups showed deterioration only in the 'Story Recall' and Trail Making part A' tests and showed the fewest number of tests with significant deterioration. It was also these patients who had lowest BDI scores.

We have seen then that when MS patients are about to develop severe brain damage they describe general depressive rather than specific cognitive complaints. When the damage is very advanced, they cease to complain. This leads us to draw conclusions which are perhaps provocative:

(1) When MS patients complain of depressive symptoms, it can be an indication of severe progression of brain damage.

(2) The connection between MS and depression described in the literature is an indication that MS patients often suffer from cognitive impairment.

If our contention is correct, it means that other forms of therapy should be offered to the MS patient and his family. If cognitive dysfunction is camouflaged as slight depressive symptoms, then it must be assumed that the patient will be undergoing personality changes which for the family are difficult to understand, and work problems due to lack of overall comprehension, forgetfulness, reduced work speed, and so on. The least we should do for these patients is to explain to them and their family how the disease can develop so that they know what to expect and understand what is happening to them.

The question then arises—and to this we have no answer—'what possibility is there for cognitive rehabilitation?' It is obvious that this aspect requires greater investigation in this particular patient group.

Acknowledgements—This work was supported by Fonden for Scleroseramte på Fyn and the Danish Multiple Sclerosis Society.

References

1 Schiffer, R. B., Caine, E. D., Bamford, K. A. & Levey, S. (1983): Depressive episodes in patients with multiple sclerosis. *Am. J. Psychiatry* **140**, 1498–1500.

2 Schiffer, R. B., Wineman, N. M. & Weitkamp, L. R. (1986): Association between bipolar affection disorder and multiple sclerosis. *Am. J. Psychiatry* **143**, 94–95.

3 Schiffer, R. B. & Barbigian, H. M. (1986): Behavioural disorders in multiple sclerosis, temporal lobe epilepsy, and amyotrophic lateral sclerosis. An epidemiological study. *Arch. Neurol.* **41**, 1067–1069.

4 Schiffer, R. B. (1987): The spectrum of depression in multiple sclerosis. An approach for clinical management. *Arch. Neurol.* **44**, 596–599.

5 Joffe, R. T., Lippert, G. P., Gray, T. A., Sawa, G. & Horvath, Z. (1987): Mood disorder and multiple sclerosis. *Arch. Neurol.* **44**, 376–378.

6 Whitelock, F. A. & Siskind, M. M. (1980): Depression as a major symptom of multiple sclerosis. *J. Neurol. Neurosurg. Psychiatry* **43**, 861–865.

7 Bottenberg, E. H., Lurati, M., Lützenkirchen, J. & Grüninger, W (1975): Multiple Sklerose und Stimmungslage. *Archiv für Psychiatrie und Nervenkrankungen* **220**, 27–36.

8 Baretz, R. M. & Stephenson, G. R. (1981): Emotional response to multiple sclerosis. *Psychosomatics* **22**, 117–127.

9 McIvor, G. P., Riklan, M. & Reznikoff, M. (1984): Depression in multiple sclerosis as a function of both length and severity of illness, age, remissions and perceived social support. *J. Clin. Psychol.* **40**, 1028–1033.

10 Dalos, N. P., Rabins, P. V., Brooks, B. R. & O'Donnell, P. (1983): Disease activity and emotional state in multiple sclerosis. *Ann. Neurol.* **13**, 573–577.

11 Jambor, K. L. (1969): Cognitive functioning in multiple sclerosis. *Br. J. Psychiatry* **115**, 765–775.
12 Surridge, D. (1969): An investigation into some aspects of multiple sclerosis. *Br. J. Psychiatry* **115**, 749–764.
13 Lyon-Caen, O., Jouvent, R., Hauser, S., Chaunu, M. P., Benoit, N., Widlöcher, D. & Lhermitte, F. (1986): Cognitive function in recent onset demyelinating diseases. *Arch. Neurol.* **43**, 1138–1141.
14 Rao, S. M., Hammeke, T. A., McQuillen, M. P., Khatri, B. O. & Lloyd, D. (1984): Memory disturbances in chronic progressive multiple sclerosis. *Arch. Neurol.* **41**, 625–631.
15 Kurtzke, J. F. (1983): Rating neurologic impairment in multiple sclerosis. *Neurology* **33**, 1444–1452.
16 Beck, A. T., Ward, C. H., Mendelson, M., Mock, J. & Erbaugh, J. (1961): An inventory for measuring depression. *Arch. Gen. Psychiatry* **4**, 561–571.

17

PSYCHIATRIC MORBIDITY IN PATIENTS WITH CLINICALLY ISOLATED LESIONS OF THE TYPE SEEN IN MULTIPLE SCLEROSIS: A CLINICAL AND MRI STUDY

S. J. Logsdail, M. M. Callanan and M. A. Ron

The National Hospital for Nervous Diseases, Queen Square, London, UK

Summary

This study reports the psychiatric morbidity in 76 patients with clinically isolated lesions of the type seen in multiple sclerosis (optic neuritis, and brain stem and cord lesions). The presence or absence of brain pathology was investigated using magnetic resonance imaging (MRI). A group of 33 patients suffering from rheumatic and neurological conditions not known to involve the brain was used for comparison. Normative MRI data were obtained from a group of 40 normal volunteers.

Over half of the patients with the clinical presentation of single lesions had MRI abnormalities in the brain, but past and present psychiatric morbidity were similar in patients and controls and no significant associations were found between the presence of MRI abnormalities and psychiatric morbidity. The degree of social stress experienced by the patients with clinically isolated lesions appeared to be highly relevant in the causation of psychiatric symptoms.

Introduction

Mental illness in patients suffering from multiple sclerosis (MS) has received considerable attention since it was first reported a hundred years ago.[1] Depression, euphoria and disturbances of emotional expression, together with cognitive impairment, were the first and most commonly described symptoms,[2] but schizophrenic features, albeit less often, have also been reported.[3] The increased psychiatric morbidity in patients suffering from MS, when compared with controls without brain pathology, has led to the conclusion that the presence of neuropathological lesions plays an important role in causing psychiatric symptoms.[4,5] In a few cases psychiatric manifestations have been considered to be the first symptoms of the disease,[6,7] even when neurological abnormalities have been absent.

Magnetic resonance imaging (MRI) has made it possible to detect the lesions present in patients with definite MS[8] with a high degree of sensitivity. It has also allowed the study of patients with seemingly isolated lesions of the type known to occur in MS, namely optic neuritis, brain stem lesions and cord lesions. Ormerod *et al.*[9] found brain lesions in areas other than those responsible for the clinical symptoms in over half of such patients. Optic neuritis is the first manifestation of MS in about 20 percent of cases and approximately three-quarters of those with optic neuritis go on to develop definite MS.[10,11] No similar prospective studies have been performed in patients with brain stem or cord symptoms, but it appears likely that a similar proportion will develop unequivocal MS.[12]

In well established cases of MS it is often difficult to extricate the psychiatric manifestations attributable to the presence of neuropathological lesions from the psychological reactions to the limitations imposed by the disease on the patients' lives. The study of those with clinically isolated lesions, on the other hand, avoids some of these difficulties by allowing one to explore the effect of brain pathology on the mental state of patients who may have little or no physical disability. This group of patients has so far received little attention.

We describe here a systematic enquiry into the psychiatric abnormalities of a group of patients with clinically isolated lesions in whom the presence or absence of brain pathology was investigated using MRI. The results of the psychometric study of the same patients have been reported separately in Chapter 7.

Methods

Subjects

Seventy-six consecutive patients (31 men and 45 women) with clinically isolated lesions were included in the study. These are referred to as the index group. Thirty-two presented with optic neuritis, 23 with a brain stem syndrome and 21 with symptoms from a spinal cord lesion. The patients formed part of a large cohort undergoing a study of MRI abnormalities in MS at the National Hospital for Nervous Diseases, London. Their mean age was 37.4 years (range 16–61) and the diagnosis of a clinically isolated lesion was made after they had undergone extensive neurological assessment.[9] They were excluded from the study if they suffered from other systemic or neurological diseases, if they had sustained head injuries with post-traumatic amnesia of more than 24 hours, or if there was evidence of drug or alcohol abuse.

Patients were told that their symptoms were inflammatory in nature and that further attacks could occur. Given the prognostic uncertainty at this stage, the possibility that they suffered from MS was only discussed when the patients asked this question.

Two control groups were used for comparison. A physically disabled control group included 33 patients, eight of whom suffered from rheumatic conditions (rheumatoid arthritis, ankylosing spondylitis, and soft tissue disease), while the rest had neurological disease without known brain involvement (prolapsed intervertebral disc, peripheral neuropathy, muscular dystrophy, neurofibroma in a spinal root, ependymoma of the cord, cervical myelopathy due to spondylosis and spinal cord syrinx). The mean age of this group was 38.6 years (range 21–62). Physical disability was graded on a three point scale: 0 = able to walk unaided, 1 = able to walk with a stick or other walking aid, and 2 = needing a wheelchair. The overall degree of disability was similar in the index and control groups.

A second group of 40 normal volunteers (21 men and 19 women) was used to obtain normative scan data. The subjects in this group were officers in the Salvation Army who volunteered to take part in the study. Their mean age was 39.9 years (range 16–64). The exclusion criteria used for the clinically isolated lesion group were applied to all the control subjects.

Clinical assessment in the index group and physically disabled controls

Details of the previous medical history were collected in both groups. In the index group special attention was paid to the duration of the neurological symptoms and to whether the patients were in exacerbation or remission at the time of the interview. Exacerbation was defined, using the criteria of Poser *et al.*,[13] as a symptom or symptoms of neurological disturbance, with or without objective confirmation, lasting more than 24 hours.

A patient was considered to have suffered an episode of psychiatric illness in the past if he or she described a sustained abnormality in mental state resulting in either a consultation with a medical practitioner, or an incapacity to fulfil day to day activities at work or at home. The mental state at interview was assessed by one examiner (S.L.) who was aware of the diagnosis, but not of the MRI scan appearances. The Clinical Interview Schedule[14] was used for this purpose. This instrument is particularly useful for detecting neurotic types of symptomatology in patients attending hospital and includes ratings for subjective symptoms and for observed behaviour. The total score (range 0–33), as well as the individual symptom ratings, were used in the analysis and patients who scored 14 or more were considered to be psychiatric 'cases'. The Beck Depression Inventory (BDI)[15] was also administered. An attempt was made to examine the possible effects of social and other difficulties on the mental state using the Social Stress and Support Interview Schedule (SSSI), a semistructured interview which has a known high validity.[16] This interview explores areas likely to be relevant in the causation of psychiatric symptoms, namely work, finances, housing, social, marital and family circumstances. Each of these six areas was scored as follows: +1 if the patient had good support, 0 if neither support nor stress were in evidence, and −1 if it was the source of significant stress. A total score was obtained by adding the partial scores. The Mini Mental State test[17] was also administered as a brief screening for gross cognitive impairment.

A brief clinical history was obtained from the subjects in the normal control group to ascertain whether they fulfilled the inclusion criteria. The General Health Questionnaire[18] was administered in order to explore the presence of psychiatric symptoms. All the subjects in this group scored below the cut-off point of three for the 20-item form of the questionnaire.

MRI assessment

The imager used in the study was a 0.5 tesla Picker superconducting system used to form proton NMR images. The standard head receiver coil provided by the manufacturer was used. Multislice imaging protocols in the axial (transverse) plane were employed. In this way eight or 16 slices of 10 mm thickness and 2 mm interslice separation were examined. Later software improvements allowed the use of contiguous 10 mm and 5 mm slices. An imaging matrix of 128×256 pixels was used, with pixel dimensions of approximately 2.4×1.2 mm. Spin echo and inversion recovery sequences were used. The use of more than one sequence with differing dependence on T1 and T2 for generation of contrast allowed the maximum number of lesions to be detected when multislice imaging was used with each sequence.[9]

The scans were assessed by two raters unaware of the neurological and psychiatric diagnoses. Scans were only considered to be abnormal if both raters agreed about the presence of significant abnormalities. Equivocal scans, or those where there was not a unanimous decision, were classified as normal. Areas of abnormal signal measuring less than 2 mm in their longest diameter, abnormalities appearing in parts of the image affected by artefact, and areas of high signal that could represent the depths of a deep sulcus were excluded. Areas of increased signal in the frontal horns, often present in normal subjects, were only considered abnormal if they were larger than 5 mm if symmetrical, or if there was a difference of more than 2 mm between the sides. Lesions in the periventricular regions, with or without extension into the brain parenchyma, were considered separately from discrete areas of increased signal elsewhere in the brain. The periventricular rim was divided into seven regions: body of the ventricle, frontal, temporal and occipital horns, trigone, and third and fourth ventricles. Lesions in each of these areas were scored from 0 to 3 depending on the size of the lesion as measured by the penetration from the edge of the ventricle into the surrounding white matter (0 = <2 mm; 1 = 2 to 5 mm; 2 = 5 to 10 mm; 3 = >10 mm). Using the same scale, the following areas were scored for the presence of discrete lesions: brain stem, cerebellum, internal capsule, basal ganglia, frontal, parietal, temporal and occipital lobes. Reference was made to the 'multiplanar anatomy of the head and neck'[19] for delineation of these areas.

A 'periventricular' score was obtained by adding the scores of the seven periventricular areas, a 'frontal' score by adding the lesion scores of the areas around the frontal horns and those of the frontal lobes and a 'temporal' score by adding the scores of the areas surrounding the temporal horns to those of the temporal and parietal lobes. The total lesion score represented the sum of the 15 individually rated areas (from each hemisphere when appropriate). The inter-rater reliability for the two independent observers was 0.95.

MRI scans were obtained in 74 of the 76 index patients, 16 of the 33 physically disabled controls and all 40 normal controls. The MRI findings were discussed with the patients at their request, otherwise no information was provided about the results.

Statistical analysis

Differences between the groups were tested using non-parametric tests (Mann-Whitney) and the Kruskal-Wallis one way analysis of variance (ANOVA). Parametric tests of significance (t-test) and non-parametric correlations (Kendall tau) were used when appropriate. A logarithmic transformation of data was performed when required for the multivariate analysis of variance (MANOVA). The Statistical Package for Social Scientists (SPSS/PC)[20] was used for statistical analysis.

Results

Psychiatric morbidity in index patients and physically disabled controls

There were no significant differences beween the two groups in age, sex, education, marital status or social class, although there was a trend for the index patients to have more professional or skilled occupations than the controls (87 percent and 57 percent respectively). The controls had been ill for longer than the index patients (mean duration of illness 6.5 and 2.7 years respectively, $P < 0.001$), but the degree of physical disability was comparable in the two groups, with five index patients and three controls using wheelchairs and two other subjects in each group needing walking aids. Only three patients in the optic neuritis group had severe visual impairment.

More index patients scored as psychiatric 'cases' at interview than controls, and their Clinical Interview Schedule scores were higher than those of the controls, but these differences failed to reach statistical significance. Of the individual ratings, only those of

Table 1. *Psychiatric data in patients with clinically isolated lesions and disabled controls.* Results are means (s.d.)

	Patients with clinically isolated lesions (n = 76)		*Controls (n = 33)*	
CIS Score	7.1	(7.4)	4.8	(4.1)
BDI Score	6.3	(7.6)	4.6	(5.5)
SSSI Score*	3.7	(1.9)	4.3	(1.6)
MMS Score	28.7	(1.5)	28.8	(1.4)
CIS 'Cases'	10		2	

CIS—Clinical Interview Schedule. BDI—Beck Depression Inventory. SSSI—Social Stress and Support Interview. MMS—Mini Mental State

*Higher scores less stress. No significant differences between the groups.

observed histrionic behaviour differentiated significantly between the two groups, with the controls obtaining higher scores. Similarly, there were no significant differences between the two groups in the BDI scores or in the amount of social stress they were experiencing at the time of interview, although both scores were higher in the index group (Table 1).

In the index group the severity of the psychiatric symptoms at interview, as measured by the Clinical Interview Schedule score, showed a significant correlation with the degree of social stress experienced by the patients (Kendall tau = 0.33, $P<0.001$) and the duration of the neurological symptoms, and this correlation remained significant when age was controlled for ($P<0.05$). Thus, nine out of 10 patients who were considered to be psychiatric 'cases' had had neurological symptoms for more than a year. These correlations failed to reach statistical significance in the control group. There were no significant differences in the degree of psychiatric morbidity at interview or in the social stress experienced by men and women in either of the groups.

Twenty-eight index patients were interviewed during an exacerbation, while 44 were stable or recovering from their neurological disability (in four patients this information was not available). No significant differences in the Clinical Interview Schedule scores were detected between the two groups, although there was a trend for those with an exacerbation to have higher ratings of observed anxiety.

Eleven index patients (14 percent) and four controls (12 percent) had experienced episodes of psychiatric illness since the onset of their neurological or physical disability. The retrospective diagnoses using DSM–III criteria are shown on Table 2. Anxiety, affective illness and adjustment reactions were the commonest problems in both groups. Psychiatric symptoms followed the onset of clinically isolated lesions at variable intervals, but in eight out of 11 patients they occurred during the first two years, while none of the controls experienced psychiatric symptoms during this period. This difference reached statistical significance (Fisher's exact test $P<0.05$).

The duration of these episodes of psychiatric illness was also variable. Six patients in the index group were ill for between one and 6 months, while the remaining five were ill for periods varying from 9 months to 3 years. Three of these patients, all of whom received a diagnosis of affective illness, were considered to have abnormal mental states at interview. Four index patients had had more than one episode of psychiatric illness, while the rest

Table 2. *Psychiatric diagnoses (DSM–III)*

	Psychiatric illness before somatic symptoms		*Psychiatric illness after somatic symptoms*		*Psychiatric cases at interview*	
	Patients	*Controls*	*Patients*	*Controls*	*Patients*	*Controls*
Anxiety	2	0	3	0	2	0
Affective disorder	4	1	5	2	4	2
Adjustment disorder	6	2	2	2	2	0
Paranoid disorder	0	0	1	0	1	0
Eating disorder	2	0	0	0	0	0
Somatoform disorder	0	0	0	0	1	0
Childhood anxiety disorder	1	0	0	0	0	0

had been ill only once. These episodes were generally not severe—only one patient required hospital admission, two others were seen by psychiatrists as out-patients and the rest were treated by their general practitioners.

Episodes of psychiatric illness preceding neurological or physical disability were more common in the index group, occurring in fifteen patients (20 percent) as opposed to three controls (9 percent). However these differences failed to reach statistical significance. The retrospective diagnoses are shown in Table 2. Six index patients had psychiatric symptoms within the 3 years preceding the onset of neurological manifestations, with three of them becoming psychiatrically ill less than 12 months before the neurological illness. The same was the case for two physically disabled controls. For the rest of the subjects, the interval between the onset of psychiatric and physical symptomatology in both groups ranged between 3 and 28 years.

The type and severity of the psychiatric symptoms preceding or following the onset of the primary illness were similar in both groups, but it would appear that those whose psychiatric symptoms pre-dated the neurological disorder were a different group from those who became ill later. Thus, only three out of 15 index patients whose psychiatric symptoms occurred before the neurological disturbances became psychiatrically ill later, or had abnormal states at the time of interview, and in all of them the psychiatric symptoms remitted for long periods of time.

Psychotic symptomatology was uncommon. One control subject had a brief hypomanic episode 3 years before the prolapse of an intervertebral disc and one index patient experienced continuous mild paranoid symptoms (morbid jealousy) over a period of 5 years in addition to recurrent depressive episodes which in turn aggravated the severity of the paranoid symptoms.

No gross cognitive impairment was observed in either group, and all the subjects scored above the cut-off point of 23 on the Mini Mental State test.

Psychiatric morbidity in the index patient subgroups

Patients with optic neuritis, brain stem and cord syndromes did not differ in age, duration of neurological symptoms or frequency of psychiatric illness preceding or following the onset of the neurological manifestation. However, significant group differences in their mental states were present at the time of interview (Table 3), with optic neuritis patients obtaining significantly lower Clinical Interview Schedule scores than the other two groups. These differences were also reflected in the number of patients whose scores were above the cut-off point for 'caseness' in each group, with only one optic neuritis patient reaching this level. Significant group differences were also observed in the individual symptom scores;

Table 3. *Psychiatric morbidity in the subgroups with clinically isolated lesions*

	Optic neuritis (n = 32)	*Brain stem (n = 23)*	*Cord (n = 21)*	
CIS score (s.d.)	4.6 (4.9)*	7.9 (6.7)	10.0 (9.9)	F = 3.9
CIS cases	1	4	5	
Individual CIS ratings				
Sleep disturbance	0.41	0.54	1.50*	F = 4.9
Depressed thoughts	0.16	0.18	0.61*	F = 4.7
Subjective anxiety	0.12	0.32	0.44*	F = 4.6
Subjective depression	0.28*	0.73	0.67	F = 3.4

CIS = Clinical Interview Schedule
*Group scores significantly different $P < 0.05$.

thus the cord group obtained significantly higher ratings for sleep disturbance, depressive thoughts and observed anxiety.

Higher ratings of subjective depression were present in both cord and brain stem patients when compared with the optic neuritis group. The degree of social stress and the BDI scores were similar in the three groups.

Nine patients with clinically isolated lesions were receiving steroids at the time of the interview, but their Clinical Interview Schedule scores did not differ from the rest of the group.

MRI differences between index patients and controls

Minor MRI abnormalities were present in five out of the 40 normal controls. In all five cases a narrow periventricular rim of increased signal was observed and, in addition, three of them had one other lesion less than 5 mm in diameter in brain parenchyma. The frequency and type of MRI abnormalities were similar in the physically disabled control group, in which two out of 16 patients were considered to have abnormal scans. One of these two patients scored within the 'caseness' range at psychiatric interview and suffered from a prolapsed intervertebral disc. The other was psychiatrically normal and had an isolated neurofibroma of a spinal root. The mean ages of the normal and physically disabled controls with abnormal scans were significantly higher than those of the remainder of the group (means 52 and 38.2 years respectively).

MRI scans were completed in 74 index patients and abnormalities were detected in 51 (69 percent). Increased periventricular signal was the commonest abnormality and was

Table 4. *MRI abnormalities in patients with clinically isolated lesions and controls*

	Patients with clinically isolated lesions (n = 74)	*Disabled controls (n = 16)*	*Normal controls (n = 40)*
Abnormal scans (%)	51 (69)	2 (12.5)	4 (12.5)
MRI lesion score (s.d.)	7.75 (10.07)	0.75 (1.43)	0.52 (2.08)
			F = 13.78*

*$p < 0.001$

present in 47 out of the 51 patients. The areas most frequently involved were those adjacent to the trigones and bodies of the lateral ventricles, followed by the frontal periventricular areas (80 percent and 72 percent respectively in those with abnormal scans). Thirty patients with periventricular lesions had, in addition, discrete lesions elsewhere in the brain, while discrete lesions without periventricular abnormalities were observed in only two patients. There were no significant differences between the total lesion score or the percentage of abnormal scans when the three subgroups of index patients were compared, although there was a non-significant trend for the optic neuritis patients to have a lower lesion score. These minor differences were due to the lower lesion scores in the right internal capsule and left basal ganglia in the optic neuritis group. On the other hand, the lesion score of the index group as a whole was significantly different from those of the two control groups.

Clinical correlates of MRI abnormalities in index patients

Five out of the 51 index patients who had abnormal MRI scans were considered to be 'cases' at interview, as were three out of the 23 patients with normal scans (Table 5). These differences were not statistically significant. No significant correlations were found between the total Clinical Interview Schedule scores and the frontal, temporal, periventricular or total lesion scores. Equally, no significant correlations were found between the various lesion scores and the individual symptoms rated by the Clinical Interview Schedule, with the exception of greater sleep disturbance in those with higher periventricular scores (Kendall tau = 0.20, $P<0.05$) or higher temporal scores (Kendall tau = 0.27, $P<0.01$). On the other hand, the severity of psychiatric symptoms at interview, as reflected by the Clinical Interview Schedule scores, and the degree of social stress were significantly higher in the group where no MRI abnormalities were in evidence.

A subgroup of 23 patients was identified who exhibited psychiatric symptoms at the time of interview, or who had been psychiatrically ill after the neurological symptoms became apparent. No significant differences in total lesion scores, or in frontal, temporal or periventricular scores were found between these patients and the rest of the group.

Temporal scores were significantly lower in the 15 patients whose psychiatric symptoms had preceded the onset of neurological abnormalities when compared with the rest of the group (Mann-Whitney $z = -3$, $P<0.005$), although the other lesion scores did not differ significantly.

To explore further the possible associations between the psychiatric morbidity observed at interview and other clinical and MRI variables, a multivariate analysis of variance (MANOVA) was performed using the Clinical Interview Schedule score as the dependent variable (Table 6). The other variables entered in the analysis were selected on empirical grounds as being likely to have a role in the genesis of psychiatric symptoms. Age, duration of illness, physical disability, exacerbation status, degree of social stress and total lesion

Table 5. *MRI/psychiatric correlations in the clinically isolated lesion group (n = 74)*

	Abnormal scan (n = 51)	*Normal scan (n = 74)*	
CIS cases	5	3	
CIS score (s.d.)	6.1 (7.4)	7.1 (5.8)	$z = -2.2$*
SSSI score (s.d.)†	3.9 (2.0)	3.2 (1.8)	$z = 2.3$*

*$p<0.05$ (Mann-Whitney)
†Higher scores, less stress

Table 6. *Correlates of psychiatric morbidity in patients with clinically isolated lesions: multivariate analysis of variance (n = 68)*

CIS score, dependent variable	*Mean square*	*F*	*Significance*
Social stress score	1093.8	34.8	< 0.0001
Degree of physical disability	7.8	0.2	0.62
Exacerbation status	0.4	0.01	0.91
Duration of illness	25.6	0.8	0.37
Age	93.9	3.0	0.09
Total lesion score	5.0	0.2	0.69

CIS = Clinical Interview Schedule

score were thus chosen as independent variables. A significant association was found between the severity of the psychiatric symptoms and the degree of social stress, and a non-significant trend was found between increasing age and the severity of the psychiatric symptoms. However, no significant associations were found between the severity of the psychiatric symptoms and the presence of MRI abnormalities.

Discussion

We report here the first systematic study of psychiatric morbidity in a group of patients presenting with clinically isolated lesions of the type often encountered in MS, in whom the presence of brain pathology had been documented using MRI. The results of the study suggest that psychiatric morbidity, although more often encountered in these subjects, was not significantly greater than in a control group of patients matched for disability, but without known brain pathology.

The choice for a control group for this kind of study is fraught with difficulties, for it is practically impossible to match the subjects for all the relevant features of the disease. The control subjects in our study had been ill for longer than the index subjects and pain was frequently a feature of their illness. Given these differences, the trend towards greater frequency and severity of psychiatric abnormalities in those with clinically isolated lesions might reflect an increased tendency to develop psychiatric disorders in these patients, perhaps as a result of the presence of brain pathology. The prevalence of psychiatric morbidity at interview in the index patients (13 percent) is slightly lower than that reported by Goldberg & Blackwell[21] among general practice attenders (20 percent), and much lower than that found in acute neurological admissions (43 percent) by Bridges & Goldberg[22] using the General Health Questionnaire. These results alone would suggest that in the present sample brain pathology can have played only a limited role in causing psychiatric symptoms.

The low frequency of psychiatric morbidity in these patients also contrasts with the much higher rates reported in patients with definite MS,[5,23,24] although the type of symptomatology, principally a mixture of features of anxiety and depression, is similar in the two groups. Important differences are nevertheless present, namely, no patients with clinically isolated lesions were found to be euphoric using the strict operational criteria of the Clinical Interview Schedule, and psychotic symptoms were also very rare. In striking contrast with the findings of Dalos *et al.*[25] of increased psychiatric symptomatology during relapses in patients with definite MS, few similar changes were found in this study. Doubtless, these differences are due to the more extensive brain pathology and greater physical disability present in definite MS.

The difference in psychiatric morbidity in the three subgroups with clinically isolated lesions was an unexpected finding, given that the duration of symptoms and degree of demonstrable brain pathology were similar across the groups and that none of the subjects suffered from chronic progressive symptoms. The possibility remains that patients with optic neuritis had less severe symptoms and were less often aware that they might suffer from MS than those with cord or brain-stem syndromes, and this may have resulted in less psychiatric morbidity.

Psychiatric illness, and in particular depression, has been considered in some cases to be the first manifestation of demyelination.[6,7] Although this may occur in rare cases, with severe and widespread pathology, the results of this study add little support to this possibility. The incidence of psychiatric illness before the onset of somatic symptoms was not significantly greater in these patients than in the controls. Moreover, most of the patients with clinically isolated lesions who had had psychiatric symptoms before their neurological illness remained well afterwards, suggesting that factors other than brain pathology might have been at work during their early psychiatric illness. In addition, these patients exhibited fewer MRI abnormalities in the temporal lobes than the rest of the group, and an association between pathology in this area and psychiatric morbidity in MS patients has recently been reported.[26]

Among the various factors which could have played a part in the causation of psychiatric symptoms at the time of the study, the degree of social stress and lack of support experienced by the patients appear to be the most relevant. This is in keeping with the findings of Mann *et al.*[27] in patients attending their general practitioners, and highlighted the importance of environmental factors, whether or not independent of the disease process, in the genesis of psychiatric symptoms. The fact that some patients were aware that they might suffer from MS did not appear to have a significant effect on the overall psychiatric morbidity. Steroids, on the other hand, do not appear to have been a contributory factor in precipitating abnormal mental states in patients with clinically isolated lesions. The contributory factors to the psychiatric morbidity of the physically disabled controls were less clear-cut and this may have been due to the greater heterogeneity of this group, which included patients with benign conditions unlikely to recur or cause significant or prolonged degrees of distress, together with others in whom the disease ran a more protracted course allowing for greater chances of psychological adaptation.

The MRI abnormalities in patients suffering from clinically isolated lesions have recently been reported by Ormerod *et al.*[9] Suffice it to say here that the MRI abnormalities are similar in type and distribution to those seen in definite MS, but the lesion scores obtained in the two groups differed significantly. Thus, while the highest score obtained by patients with clinically isolated lesions was 9, patients with definite MS obtained ratings up to 42 in Ormerod's series, which used the same scoring system as this study.

MRI abnormalities in healthy volunteers have also been described, in particular increased periventricular signal in patients over the age of 60 years.[28] The origin of these abnormalities remains uncertain, but the possibility that they may be due to cerebral involvement in childhood exanthemata or to occult vascular disease has been put forward.[9] The control patients with MRI abnormalities in this study were significantly older than the rest of the group, but there were no other obvious explanations for the presence of lesions.

For practical reasons it was not possible to scan all the physically disabled patients included in this study, but the similar frequency of MRI abnormalities in the normal and physically disabled controls suggests that our selection criteria were affective in excluding those in whom brain pathology may have been an integral part of the rheumatic or neurological conditions that they suffered from. As expected, the extent and frequency of detectable brain pathology was much greater in the index group. The lack of positive correlations between the presence of physchiatric abnormalities and lesions detected by

MRI was disappointing, although not totally unexpected, given the overall low psychiatric morbidity of these patients and the greater severity of social stress experienced by those without MRI abnormalities. In particular, these results failed to confirm the findings of Horner *et al.*[26] who reported increased psychiatric symptomatology in definite MS patients with demonstrable temporal lobe pathology. In our sample only a modest correlation with insomnia occurred and little weight can be given to this isolated finding.

The discrepancy between the clinical manifestation of MS and the extent of neuropathological lesions encountered at autopsy is well known and cases of benign or silent MS have often been reported.[29-31] Several reasons may account for this. Mild symptoms may be forgotten by the patient, and neural factors, such as the speed of development of the lesion and the 'redundancy' within some pathways that require a critical level of damage before function is impaired, may be important.[32] However, the possibility remains that the appropriate assessment to detect the clinical manifestations of the lesions has not been performed.

Subtle memory changes in a handful of patients with optic neuritis have been reported by Lyon-Caen *et al.*,[33] and detailed psychometric testing in our patients[13] also suggests that mild cognitive impairment may be a more reliable indicator of the presence of brain pathology. On the other hand the results of this study suggest that psychiatric symptoms are not the direct clinical counterparts of the lesions detected by MRI. The possibility still remains that only lesions affecting specific cerebral systems (eg the limbic system) may have a bearing on the causation of psychiatric symptoms, and more refined methods of clinico-anatomical correlation will need to be used to explore this further.

Finally, in view of the paucity of psychopathology in these patients, caution is required when evaluating the role of minor structural brain abnormalities in those suffering from major psychiatric illness.

Acknowledgements – We are indebted to the members of the MRI research group at the National Hospital for Nervous Diseases and to the MS Society for providing the MRI scanner. We are also grateful to Professor W. A. Lishman and Professor W. I. McDonald who made helpful comments on the manuscript and to Mrs T. Guise for typing it. Finally, our thanks are due to all the patients who took part in the study and their consultants who allowed us to approach them. The study was supported by a grant from the Medical Research Council.

This chapter is based on an article published in *Psychological Medicine*, 1988, **18**, 355–364. Permission to reprint it has been received from Cambridge University Press.

References

1 Charcot, J. M. (1877): *Lectures on the Diseases of the Nervous System*. New Sydenham Society: London.

2 Cottrell, S. S. & Wilson, S. A. K. (1926): The affective symptomatology of disseminated sclerosis. *J. Neurol. Psychopathol.* **7**, 1–30.

3 Davison, K. & Bagley, C. R. (1969): Schizophrenia-like psychoses associated with organic disorders of the central nervous system: a review of the literature. In *Current problems in neuropsychiatry*, ed R. N. Herrington, pp 113–184. Ashford, Kent: Headley.

4 Schiffer, R. B., Caine, E. D., Bamford, K. A. & Levy, S. (1983): Depressive symptoms in patients with multiple sclerosis. *Am. J. Psychiatry* **140**, 1498–1500.

5 Rabins, P. V., Brooks, B. R., O'Donnell, P., Pearlson, G. D., Moberg, P., Jubelt, B., Coyle, P., Dalos, N. & Folstein, M. F. (1986): Structural brain correlates of emotional disorder in multiple sclerosis. *Brain* **109**, 585–597.

6 Matthews, W. B. (1979): Multiple sclerosis presenting with acute remitting psychiatric symptoms. *J. Neurol. Neurosurg. Psychiatry* **42**, 859–863.

7 Whitlock, F. A. & Siskind, M. M. (1980): Depression as a major symptom of multiple sclerosis. *J. Neurol. Neurosurg. Psychiatry* **43**, 861–865.
8 Young, I. R., Hall, A. S., Pallis, C. A., Legg, N. J., Bydder, G. M. & Steiner, R. E. (1981): Nuclear magnetic resonance imaging of the brain in multiple sclerosis. *Lancet* **ii**, 1063–1066.
9 Ormerod, I. E. C., Miller, D. H., McDonald, W. I., du Boulay, E. P. G. H., Rudge, P., Kendall, B. E., Moseley, I. F., Johnson, G., Tofts, P. S., Halliday, A. M., Bronstein, A. M., Scaravilli, F., Harding, A. E., Barnes, D. & Zilkha, K. J. (1987): The role of NMR imaging in the assessment of multiple sclerosis and isolated neurological lesions: A quantitative study. *Brain* **110**, 1579–1616.
10 McDonald, W. I. (1983): The significance of optic neuritis. *Trans. Ophthalmol. Soc. UK* **103**, 230–246.
11 Francis, D. A., Compston, D. A. S., Batchelor, J. R. & McDonald, W. I. (1987): A reassessment of the risk of multiple sclerosis developing in patients with optic neuritis after extended follow-up. *J. Neurol. Neurosurg. Psychiatry* **50**, 758–765.
12 McDonald, W. I. & Silberberg, D. H. (1986): The diagnosis of multiple sclerosis. In *Multiple sclerosis*, eds W. I. McDonald & D. H. Silberberg, pp 1–10. London: Butterworths.
13 Poser, C. M., Paty, D. W., Scheinberg, L., McDonald, W. I., Davis, S. A., Ebers, G. C. I., Johnson, K. P., Sibley, W. A., Silberberg, D. H. & Tourtelotte, W. W. (1983): New diagnostic criteria for multiple sclerosis: Guidelines for research protocols. *Ann. Neurol.* **13**, 227–231.
14 Goldberg, D. P., Cooper, B., Eastwood, M. R., Kedward, H. B. & Shepherd, M. (1970): A standardized psychiatric interview for use in community surveys. *Br. J. Prev. Soc. Med.* **24**, 18–23.
15 Beck, A. T., Ward, C. H., Mendelson, M., Mock, J. & Erbaugh, J. (1961): An inventory for measuring depression. *Arch. Gen. Psychiatry* **4**, 561–571.
16 Jenkins, R., Mann, A. H. & Belsey, E. (1981): Design and use of a short interview to assess social stress and support in research and clinical settings. *Soc. Sci. Med.* **151**, 195–203.
17 Folstein, M. F., Folstein, S. E. & McHugh, P. R. (1975): 'Mini Mental State'. A practical method for grading the cognitive state of patients for the clinician. *J. Psychiatr. Res.* **12**, 189–198.
18 Goldberg, D. P. (1972): *The detection of psychiatric illness by questionnaire*. London: Oxford University Press.
19 Palacios, E., Fine, M. & Haughton, V. M. (1980): *Multiplanar anatomy of the head and neck for computer tomography*. New York: John Wiley.
20 Norusis, M. J. (1986): *SPSS/PC for the IBM PC/XT/AT*. Chicago: SPSS.
21 Goldberg, D. P. & Blackwell, B. (1970): Psychiatric illness in general practice. A detailed study using a new method of case identification. *Br. Med. J.* **ii**, 439–443.
22 Bridges, K. W. & Goldberg, D. P. (1984): Psychiatric illness in patients with neurological disorders: patients' views on discussion of emotional problems with neurologists. *Br. Med. J.* **289**, 656–658.
23 Surridge, D. (1969): An investigation into some psychiatric aspects of multiple sclerosis. *Br. J. Psychiatry* **115**, 749–764.
24 Schiffer, R. B. & Barbigian, H. M. (1984): Behavioural disorders in multiple sclerosis, temporal lobe epilepsy and amyotrophic lateral sclerosis. *Arch. Neurol.* **41**, 1067–1069.
25 Dalos, N. P., Rabins, P. V., Brooks, B. R. & O'Donnell, P. (1983): Disease activity and emotional state in multiple sclerosis. *Ann. Neurol.* **13**, 573–577.
26 Horner, W. G., Hurwitz, T., Li, D. K. B., Palmer, M. & Paty, D. W. (1987): Temporal lobe involvement in multiple sclerosis patients with psychiatric disorders. *Arch. Neurol.* **44**, 187–190.
27 Mann, A. H., Jenkins, R. & Belsey, E. (1981): The twelve month outcome of patients with neurotic illness in general practice. *Psychol. Med.* **11**, 535–550.
28 Brant-Zawadski, M., Fein, G., Van Dyke, C., Kiernan, R., Davenport, L. & de Groot, J. (1985): MR imaging of the aging brain: patchy white matter lesion in dementia. *Am. J. Neuroradiol.* **6**, 675–682.
29 Fog, T., Hyllested, K. & Andersen, S. R. (1972): A case of benign multiple sclerosis with autopsy. *Acta Neurol. Scand. Suppl.* **51**, 369–370.
30 Ghatak, N. R., Hirano, A., Lutmaer, H. & Zimmerman, H. M. (1974): Asymptomatic demyelinated plaque in the spinal cord. *Arch. Neurol.* **30**, 484–486.

31 Gilbert, J. J. & Sadler, M. (1983): Unsuspected multiple sclerosis. *Arch. Neurol.* **40**, 533–536.
32 McDonald, W. I. (1986): The pathophysiology of multiple sclerosis. In *Multiple sclerosis*, eds W. I. McDonald & D. H. Silberberg, pp 112–133. London: Butterworths.
33 Lyon-Caen, O., Jouvent, R., Hauser, S., Chau Nu, M. P., Benoit, N., Widlöcher, D. & Lhermitte, F. (1986): Cognitive function in recent onset demyelinating diseases. *Arch. Neurol.* **43**, 1138–1141.

VII

MENTAL DISORDER AND A GENETIC AETIOLOGY

18

MULTIPLE SCLEROSIS AND AFFECTIVE DISORDER: FAMILY HISTORY, SEX AND HLA-DR ANTIGENS

Randolph B. Schiffer*, Lowell R. Weitkamp†§, N. Margaret Wineman‡ and Sally Guttormsen†

**Departments of Psychiatry, Neurology, and Center for Brain Research, †Division of Genetics, §Department of Pediatrics, and ‡Department of Psychiatric Nursing, University of Rochester Medical Center, 601 Elmwood Avenue, Rochester, New York 14642, USA*

Summary

In order to investigate a possible genetic aetiology underlying the clinical association between multiple sclerosis (MS) and affective disorder, we studied 56 MS patients for psychiatric and genetic (family history, sex and HLA-DR) characteristics. The 2:1 ratio of females to males expected for MS patients was observed in this sample (40:16), but the excess of females occurred entirely among the 31 MS patients with major affective disorder (27 female:4 male). Bipolar MS probands had significantly more relatives with affective disorder or MS than did unipolar MS probands. HLA-DR antigen frequencies in MS patients categorized by type and family history of affective disorder provide a suggestion that it may be possible to validate such clustering of patients.

We conclude that sex and other genetic factors are related to the affective symptomatology in MS and emphasize the importance of psychiatric evaluation of these patients.

Introduction

We have recently reported an association between bipolar affective disorder and multiple sclerosis (MS) within the population of Monroe County, New York.[1] Since that epidemiological study included no investigation of mechanisms by which such an association might occur, we report here the results of a follow-up genetic study. The study included nine of the original 10 patients, as well as 47 additional MS patients with or without major affective disorder.

Although there is increased familial occurrence of MS as well as affective disorder, no simple genetic pattern for either disease is apparent. Both MS and unipolar disorder are more common in females, whereas bipolar disorder shows a smaller female preponderance.[2-4] Twin studies indicate that MS disease concordance may approach 26–30 percent for monozygotic twins, while it is 10–13 percent or possibly as low as 2–3 percent for dizygotic twins.[5,6] In contrast to an 11–14 percent concordance rate for either bipolar or unipolar disorder in dizygotic twins, the concordance rate for bipolar disorder in monozygotic twins is as high as 70 percent and for unipolar disorder possibly 40 percent.[7]

Multiple studies have confirmed an association of certain HLA (human leucocyte antigen) alleles with MS in patients of Northwest European origin.[8-17] These genes control the expression of surface antigens on immunocompetent cells, and are implicated in vulnerability to many diseases that have an autoimmune character. The HLA system is determined by genes at several loci or sites on the short arm of chromosome 6. Two of several alternative alleles are possible for any individual at each locus. Caucasian MS patients demonstrate an increased frequency of the alleles A3, B7, and DR2, with DR2 showing the strongest association. However, DR2 is present in only half of MS patients. Other deviations from random gene frequencies that have been reported among MS patients include increased frequency of A1, A3, A9, B8 and DR3, and decreased frequency of A2, B12, B15, Bw22, B40, DR1, DRw6 and DR7.[8,11] The effect of HLA genes or genes in the HLA region of chromosome 6 on susceptibility to MS may be mediated by the sex of the patient.[18]

For psychiatric diseases in general, and for the affective disorders in particular, it has proven more difficult to identify such relationships to HLA genes. There have been reports of patterns of assortment of HLA alleles that are not random in at least some families with affective disorders.[19-22] Other investigators have not observed a relationship to genes on chromosome 6.[23-28]

We report here our results of family studies and of HLA typing of MS patients with and without major affective disorders. The loci typed included HLA-A, B, C, DR and DQ. Previous studies of HLA antigens in affective disorders have generally not included typing for HLA-DR or DQ antigens.

Methods

Clinical selection

For the past 3 years, all patients in the University of Rochester MS Clinic with definite multiple sclerosis by research criteria[29] have been screened for possible entry into this study. Approximately 350 patients are followed in this clinic, and all are encouraged to attend at least once per year. Patients who showed evidence of possible affective disturbance during their clinic visits were referred to the investigators for definitive psychiatric evaluation. Selected MS patients who seemed never to have experienced emotional disturbance were also referred to the investigators as potential controls. Referred MS patients were interviewed by one investigator (NMW), using the Schedule for Affective Disorders and Schizophrenia (SADS-L),[30] and psychiatric diagnoses were made in accordance with the Research Diagnostic Criteria (RDC).[31] From among these interviewed patients, 40 with very definite diagnoses—11 bipolar, 16 unipolar, and 13 with no affective disturbance—were selected for this study. Nine of the bipolar MS patients have been reported in a previous study.[3] In order to increase the number of bipolar MS subjects, three additional patients were studied at the University of Western Ontario, London, Ontario through the courtesy of Dr. George Ebers, and one was seen at the Dent Neurologic Institute, Buffalo,

New York through the courtesy of Dr. Lawrence Jacobs. These four subjects were interviewed using the SADS-L. All of the above 44 subjects were given a standardized family history interview and were typed for HLA antigens. An additional 12 MS patients who had *little* affective symptomatology based on the SADS-L interview, but who were not completely free of depressive symptomatology were judged not to have major affective disorder and were typed for HLA antigens. They were selected in order to increase the number of control (no affective disorder) MS subjects typed for HLA antigens.

Family history

A family history of either affective disorders or MS among family members was obtained by standardized interview from the 44 MS probands, as indicated above. In the interview, questions were asked concerning possible affective disorders for all first degree relatives, as well as for cousins, nieces, aunts, uncles, and grandparents. For a relative to be considered 'positive' for an affective disorder, a history of diagnosis by a psychiatrist, a suicide, or a clear description of the affective episode with diagnosis in accordance with RDC was required. A relative was considered positive for MS if the diagnosis had been made by a neurologist. A detailed listing of the extent of information available from the family history for each of the 44 families interviewed is given in Appendix I.

Genetic typing

Blood samples from the 56 subjects were collected by antecubital venepuncture in Vacutainers containing acid citrate dextrose (formulation A, National Institute of Health) and typed for HLA antigens within 36 hours. HLA typing was performed using the standard NIH microlymphocytotoxicity test, but with fluorescein diacetate and ethidium bromide as counter stains.[21] HLA-A, B, and C typing was performed on T-lymphocytes, and HLA-DR and DQ typing was performed on B-lymphocytes separated on nylon wool columns.[32] All subjects were typed for 16 HLA-A specificities (A1, A2, A3, A11, A23, A24, A25, A26, A28, A29, A30, A31, A32, Aw33, Aw34, and Aw36), 27 HLA-B specificities (B7, B8, B13, B14, B18, B27, Bw22, B35, B37, B38, B39, Bw41, Bw42, B44, B45, Bw47, B49, Bw50, B51, Bw52, Bw53, Bw57, Bw58, Bw60, Bw61, Bw62, and Bw63), 4 HLA-C specificities (Cw1, Cw2, Cw3, and Cw4), and 9 HLA-DR specificities (DR1, DR2, DR3, DR4, DR5, DRw6, DR7, DRw8, and DRw9). All subjects were also typed for Bw4 and Bw6 and all but two subjects were typed for DRw52 and DRw53. Twenty-four subjects were typed for HLA-DQw1, DQw2, and DQw3 and another 28 subjects were typed for DQw1 and DQw3 only. A few subjects were typed for HLA-Cw5, Cw6, Cw7, and Cw8. Two subjects whose cells reacted with both Bw57 and Bw58 antisera were typed as HLA-B17.

Results and discussion

Family history study

Among the 56 MS patients, 15 had bipolar disorder, 16 had unipolar disorder, 13 had no affective disorder, and 12 probably had no affective disorder. A family history of MS and affective disorder was obtained for each of the 44 probands for whom there was a detailed investigation and definite conclusion with respect to affective status. A summary of results based on the family history data is shown in Table 1. A positive family

Table 1. *Family history status of 44 MS probands.*

Family history of:	*Number of MS probands according to affective status* Bipolar	Unipolar	No disorder
MS and bipolar disorder	3		
MS and unipolar disorder	1		
MS, no affective disorder			1
Bipolar, no MS	4		
Unipolar, no MS	2	1	1
No MS or affective disorder	5	15	11
Total	15	16	13

history of MS or affective disorder is shown only for those probands who had a relative with an unequivocally positive history. Ten of the 15 bipolar probands had a positive family history for affective disorder, whereas one of the 16 unipolar and two of the 13 patients without affective disorder had such a history. In addition, all seven of the probands who had a relative with bipolar disorder occurred in the group of 15 bipolar MS probands. The increased frequency of bipolar MS probands with a family history of affective disorder is significant when compared with unipolar MS probands (χ_1^2 with Yates correction = 9.9, $P<0.005$) or with all non-bipolar MS probands (χ_1^2 with Yates correction = 14.9, $P<0.001$). The family history data should, of course, be treated cautiously since they are limited by the size of the family, knowledge of the informants, and extent of inquiry. However, our results are consistent with other studies showing a greater incidence of affective disorder among relatives of bipolar probands as compared with unipolar probands. The results suggest that genetic susceptibility to bipolar disorder in bipolar MS patients may be similar in some respect to that in bipolar patients without MS.

Five of the 44 MS probands had relatives with MS. Four of these probands were from the bipolar MS proband group and one was from the group of MS probands with no affective disorder. All four of the bipolar MS probands who had a relative with MS had other relatives with affective disorder, and in one case the relative with MS also had affective disorder. Although the number of cases reported here is small, these coincidences, together with our previous report of an increase over random expectation in the co-occurrence of bipolar disorder and MS in the same patient,[1] suggests that some genes or combinations of genes may increase susceptibility to both MS and bipolar affective disorder.

Sex and diagnostic category

The sex of each of the 56 subjects is shown in Appendix II according to the four diagnostic groupings. Three of the 15 bipolar MS probands and one of the 16 unipolar MS probands were male. In contrast, six of the 13 MS probands with no affective disorder and six of the 12 probands with probably no affective disorder were male. For analysis of the sex distribution, we included the 12 patients who failed to meet criteria for affective disturbance, but who were not completely free of affective symptomatology by interview, in the category of no affective disorder. The decreased frequency of males among MS patients with definite affective disorder as compared with MS patients without definite affective disorder was significant (χ_1^2 with Yates correction = 6.7, $P<0.01$). It is of interest that the well-documented overall 2:1 increased incidence of MS in females compared with males[18] was accounted for in our subject population entirely by MS patients with affective disorder (27 female of 31 subjects).

Since affective disorder with MS may in a sense be considered more 'severe' than affective disorder without MS, we have also examined the sex distribution among all 34 affectively ill relatives in the 12 families with an affectively ill member (Table 1). One relative, a male, had both bipolar disorder and MS, four males and seven females had bipolar disorder, and seventeen males and five females had unipolar disorder (cf. Appendix II). Taking into account the 11 probands with affective disorder (Tables 1 and 2), the proportion of affected males and females in these familial cases was equal (23:22). However, the extent or at least the type of illness corresponded to the sex of the person. Among the 45 family members, two males and nine females had bipolar disorder and MS, one female had unipolar disorder and MS, four males and seven females had bipolar disorder without MS, and 17 males and five females had unipolar disorder without MS. Thus affective disorder with MS was primarily a female disease whereas in these same families unipolar disorder without MS was principally a male disorder. The latter observation is striking because unipolar affective disorder is overall more common in females; even with a null hypothesis of no sex difference in the frequency of unipolar disorder among unipolar patients in these families, the increased frequency of males was significant (χ_1^2 with Yates correction $= 5.5$, $P < 0.025$).

HLA, Diagnostic category, and family history of affective disorder

The HLA types of each of the 56 probands are shown in Appendix II. HLA-DR antigen frequencies in each of the four diagnostic groupings, together with antigen frequencies calculated from a published control group, are summarized in Table 2. The increase over random in the frequencies of DR2 and DR3 antigens reported for MS patients by others[8,11] was observed in our total sample of 56 patients. The increased frequency of DR2 and DR3 antigens was offset principally by a decreased frequency of DR5 and DR7. A decreased frequency of DR7 in MS patients has been noted previously.[11]

Since the number of MS subjects in each of the three major groups—bipolar, unipolar, and no affective disorder—is small in relation to the number of HLA-DR antigens typed, we have made no tests of statistical significance for HLA-DR antigen frequency differences among groups. However, we do note that the increased frequency of DR2 occurred in patients with no affective disorder (0.48) or with bipolar affective disorder (0.47), whereas the frequency of DR2 in MS patients with unipolar disorder (0.31) was similar to the frequency in controls (0.30). Further, MS patients with no affective disorder or with bipolar affective disorder were more different from controls in the frequency of other DR antigens than were the MS patients with unipolar disorder. Specifically, DR5 and DR7 were the antigens that were most decreased in frequency in the patients without affective disorder; DR1 and DR4 were most decreased in the patients with bipolar disorder.

Since 10 of the 15 bipolar MS patients and only one of the unipolar MS patients had a positive family history of affective disorder, absence of DR1 and DR4 could also be a marker of the genetic susceptibility that is indicated by a positive family history of affective disorder. Thus, we have also tabulated HLA-DR antigen frequencies according to family history of affective disorder; the results are shown in Table 3 for the 31 MS probands with affective disorder. In the 11 subjects with a positive family history of affective disorder, there was an increase in DR5 and DRw6 as well as a decrease in DR1 and DR4, as compared with the 20 subjects with a negative family history of affective disorder.

Sex, HLA-DR, and family history of multiple sclerosis

The frequencies of HLA-DR antigens were very similar in males compared with females among the MS patients without affective disorder (cf. Appendix II). This is the group

Table 2. *HLA-DR antigen frequencies in 56 multiple sclerosis patients according to psychiatric diagnosis.*

	No affective disorder			*Affective disorder*						
	Definite (13)	*Probable (12)*	*Total (25)*	*Bipolar (15)*		*Unipolar (16)*		*Total (31)*	*Total MS (56)*	*Controls**
HLA-DR antigen	*No.*	*No.*	*Frequency*	*No.*	*Frequency*	*No.*	*Frequency*	*Frequency*	*Frequency*	*Frequency*
DR1	3	0	0.12	0	0.00	5	0.31	0.16	0.14	0.18
DR2	5	7	0.48	7	0.47	5	0.31	0.39	0.43	0.30
DR3	4	3	0.28	5	0.33	4	0.25	0.29	0.29	0.21
DR4	5	4	0.36	1	0.07	5	0.31	0.19	0.27	0.25
DR5	1	0	0.04	5	0.33	2	0.13	0.23	0.14	0.27
DRw6	5	4	0.36	2	0.13	2	0.13	0.13	0.23	0.22
DR7	1	1	0.08	2	0.13	2	0.13	0.13	0.11	0.23
DRw8	0	1	0.04	1	0.07	1	0.06	0.06	0.05	0.06
DRw9	0	1	0.04	0		0			0.02	0.02

*Calculated from data in Albert *et al.*[33]

Table 3. *HLA-DR antigen frequencies in 31 multiple sclerosis-affective disorder probands according to family history of affective disorder.*

	Positive family history (11)		*Negative family history (20)*		*Controls*
HLA-DR antigen	*No.*	*Frequency*	*No.*	*Frequency*	*Frequency*
DR1	0	0.00	5	0.25	0.18
DR2	5	0.45	7	0.35	0.30
DR3	3	0.27	6	0.30	0.21
DR4	0	0.00	6	0.30	0.25
DR5	4	0.36	3	0.15	0.27
DRw6	3	0.27	1	0.05	0.22
DR7	2	0.18	2	0.10	0.23
DRw8	1	0.09	1	0.05	0.06

in which the frequency of males and females was similar. For the 31 MS probands with affective disorder, of which only four were male, there was also no remarkable difference in HLA-DR frequencies between sexes. On the other hand, the four bipolar MS probands who had a family history of both MS and affective disorder (Table 1), MD021, MD035, MD030, and MD032 (Appendix II), had HLA-DR phenotypes DR5; DR2,5; DR2; and DR2,5; respectively. Based on HLA-DQ and w52/w53 typing, the subjects with the DR5 and DR2 phenotypes were probably homozygous for these antigens. Thus, the DR2 and DR5 antigens individually or jointly may be markers of high genetic risk for the phenotype of multiple sclerosis with bipolar affective disorder.

Conclusions

We envisage three general clusters of MS patients in terms of genetic characteristics. The first is a cluster of patients with a positive family history of affective disorder. The MS patients are usually female and usually have bipolar disorder. Among their relatives are persons with bipolar disorder, unipolar disorder and also occasionally MS. Strikingly, the relatives with unipolar disorder are usually male. The second cluster of MS patients are those with affective disorder and a negative family history of affective illness. The MS patients are nearly always female and usually have unipolar disorder. The third cluster of MS patients are those without affective disorder. These patients are equally likely to be female or male and usually have a negative family history of affective disorder or MS.

The HLA-DR antigen frequencies in patients in the three clusters provide preliminary, suggestive evidence that it may be possible to validate these clusters by different DR gene distributions within each group. All three clusters had an increased frequency of DR2 and DR3, consistent with the established increased frequency of these antigens in MS patients. The most likely frequency differences among the other DR antigens are for an increased frequency of DR5 and a decreased frequency of DR1 and DR4 in bipolar MS patients with a positive family history of affective disorder *vs* an increased frequency of DRw6 and a decreased frequency of DR5 in MS patients without affective disorder. These observations require testing in another sample of MS patients.

Acknowledgements—Supported by New Investigator Research Award NS-20838 from the National Institute of Neurological and Communicative Disorders and Stroke (Dr. Schiffer), and by grant RR-00044 from NIH, and grant MH-37121 from NIMH, and by grant 1-443 from the March of Dimes Birth Defects Foundation. Reprinted substantially from *Archives of Neurology* 1988; **45**: 1345–1348 with permission, American Medical Association.

References

1 Schiffer, R. B., Wineman, N. M. & Weitkamp, L. R. (1986): Association between bipolar affective disorder and multiple sclerosis. *Am. J. Psychiatry* **143**, 94–95.

2 Stewart, G. J. & Kirk, R. L. (1983): The genetics of multiple sclerosis: The HLA system and other genetic markers. In *Multiple sclerosis*, eds J. F. Hallpike, C. W. M. Adams & W. W. Tourtellotte, pp 97–128. Baltimore: Williams & Wilkins.

3 Winokur, G. & Crowe, R. R. (1983): The sex-polarity effect in affectively ill family members. *Arch. Gen. Psychiatry* **40**, 57–58.

4 Weissman, M. M. & Boyd, J. H. (1984): The epidemiology of affective disorders. *Neurobiology of mood disorders*, eds R. M. Post & J. C. Ballenger. Williams & Wilkins.

5 Spielman, R. S. & Nathanson, N. (1982): The genetics of susceptibility to multiple sclerosis. *Epidemiol. Rev.* **4**, 45–65.

6 Ebers, G. C., Bulman, D. E., Sadovnick, A. D., Paty, D. W., Warren, S., Hader, W., Murray, T. J., Seland, T. P., Duquette, P., Grey, T., Nelson, R., Nicolle, M. & Brunet, D. (1986): A population-based study of multiple sclerosis in twins. *N. Engl. J. Med.* **315**, 1638–1642.

7 Allen, M. G. (1976): Twin studies of affective illness. *Arch. Gen. Psychiatry* **33**, 1476–1478.

8 Haile, R. W., Hodge, S. E., Iselius, L. (1983): Genetic susceptibility to multiple sclerosis: a review. *Int. J. Epidemiol.* **12**, 8–16.

9 Meyer-Rienecker, H. J., Wegener, S., Hitschke, B. & Richter, K. V. (1982): Multiple sclerosis: relation between HLA haplotype A25, B18, and disease progression. *Acta Neurol. Scand.* **66**, 709–712.

10 Tiwari, J. L. *et al.* (1980): HLA and inheritance of multiple sclerosis: Linkage analysis of 72 pedigrees. *Am. J. Hum. Genet.* **32**, 103–111.

11 Madigand, M., Oger, J. J. F., Fauchet, R., Sabouraud, O. & Genetet, B. (1982): HLA profiles in multiple sclerosis suggest two forms of disease and the existence of protective haplotypes. *J. Neurol. Sci.* **53**, 519–529.

12 Ho, H. Z., Tiwari, J. L., Haile, R. W., Teraski, P. I. & Morton, N. E. (1982): HLA-linked and unlinked determinants of multiple sclerosis. *Immunogenetics* **15**, 509–517.

13 Teraski, P. I., Park, M. S., Opelz, G. & Ting, A. (1976): Multiple sclerosis and high incidence of a B lymphocyte antigen. *Science* **193**: 1245–1247.

14 Jersild, C., Bo, D., Torben, F., Platz, P. J. & Svejgzard, A. (1975): Histocompatibility determinants in multiple sclerosis. *Transplant Rev.* **22**, 148–163.

15 Stewart, G. J., McLeod, J. G., Besten, A. & Bashir, H. V. (1981): HLA family studies and multiple sclerosis: a common gene, dominantly expressed. *Human Immunol.* **3**, 13–29.

16 Ebers, G. C., Paty, D. W., Stiller, C. R., Nelson, R. F., Seland, T. P. & Larsen, B. (1982): HLA-typing in multiple sclerosis sibling pairs. *Lancet* **2**, 88–90.

17 Batchelor, J. R., Compston, A. & McDonald, W. I. (1978): The significance of the association between HLA and multiple sclerosis. *Br. Med. Bull.* **34**, 279–284.

18 Weitkamp, L. R. (1983): Multiple sclerosis susceptibility: interaction between sex and HLA. *Arch. Neurol.* **40**, 399–401.

19 Smeraldi, E., Negri, F., Melica, A. M. & Scorza-Smeraldi, R. (1978): HLA system and affective disorders: A sibship genetic study. *Tissue Antigens* **12**, 270–274.

20 Smeraldi, E. & Bellodi, L. (1981): Possible linkage between primary affective disorders susceptibility locus and HLA haplotypes. *Am. J. Psychiatry* **138**, 1232–1234.

21 Weitkamp, L. R., Stancer, H. C., Persad, E., Flood, C. & Guttormsen, S. (1981): Depressive disorders and HLA: A gene of chromosome 6 that can affect behavior. *N. Engl. J. Med.* **305**, 1301–1306.

22 Turner, W. J. & King, S. (1983): BDP_2 an autosomal dominant form of bipolar affective disorder. *Biol. Psychiatry* **18**, 63–88.

23 Targum, S. D., Gershon, E. S., Van Eerdewegh, M. & Rogentine, N. (1979): Human leukocyte antigen system not closely linked to or associated with bipolar manic-depressive illness. *Biol. Psychiatry* **14**, 615–636.

24 Johnson, G. F. S., Hunt, G. E., Robertson, S. & Doran, T. J. (1981): A linkage study of manic depressive disorders with HLA antigens, blood groups, serum proteins and red cell enzymes. *J. Affect. Dis.* **3**, 43–58.

25 Suarez, B. K. & Croughan, J. (1982): In the major histocompatibility complex linked to genes that increase susceptibility to affective disorder? A critical appraisal. *Psychiatr. Res.* **7**, 19–27.
26 Goldin, L. R., Clerget-Darpoux, F. & Gershon, E. S. (1982): Relationship of HLA to major affective disorder not supported. *Psychiatr. Res.* **7**, 29–45.
27 Suarez, B. K. & Reich, T. (1984): HLA and major affective disorders. *Arch. Gen. Psych.* **41**, 22–27.
28 Kidd, K. K., Egeland, J. A., Molthon, L., Pauls, D. L., Kruger, S. D. & Messner, K. H. (1984): Amish study IV: Genetic linkage study of pedigrees of bipolar probands. *Am. J. Psychiatry* **141**, 1042–1048.
29 Poser, C. M., Paty, D. W., Scheinberg, L. C. *et al.* (1983): New diagnostic criteria for multiple sclerosis: Guidelines for research protocols. *Ann. Neurol.* **13**, 227–231.
30 Endicott, J. & Spitzer, R. L. (1978): A diagnostic interview: The schedule for affective disorders and schizophrenia. *Arch. Gen. Psychiatry* **35**, 837–844.
31 Endicott, J. & Spitzer, R. L. (1979): Use of the research diagnostic criteria and the schedule for affective disorders and schizophrenia to study affective disorders. *Am. J. Psychiatry* **136**, 52–56.
32 Lowry, R., Goguen, J., Carpenter, C. B., Strom, T. B. & Garovoy, M. R. (1979): Improved B cell typing for HLA-DR using nylon wool enriched B lymphocyte preparations. *Tissue Antigens* **14**, 325–329.
33 Albert, E. D., Baur, M. P. & Mayr, W. R., eds (1984): *Histocompatibility testing 1984*. Berlin: Springer-Verlag, p 707.

Appendix I—Family history data
Bipolar MS group

Subject	Source of data: Pt	Source of data: Case record	Source of data: Fam	Incidence MS in family	Incidence of affective disorder in family: Negative	Incidence of affective disorder in family: Bipolar illness	Incidence of affective disorder in family: Unipolar illness	No. of male & female siblings	No. of maternal aunts & uncles	No. of paternal aunts & uncles	No. of maternal cousins male & female	No. of paternal cousins male & female	No. of nieces	No. of nephews	No. of children male & female
1	X	X		Negative			Mother	3 brothers 3 sisters	4 aunts 2 uncles	0	'many'	0	4	7	2 male
2	X	X		Negative		(Mother treated for schizophrenia)	Maternal grandfather and great grandfather suicide	2 brothers	9 aunts 3 uncles	1 aunt 1 uncle	'many'	2 male 1 female	2	0	0
3	X	X		Negative	X			1 brother 1 sister	2 uncles	2 aunts	2 male 4 female	0	0	3	0
4	X	X	Husband	Negative		Paternal aunt	Maternal uncle; son committed suicide	2 sisters	9 total (sex unknown)	6 total (sex unknown)	'many'	'many'	0	2	1 male 1 female
5	X	X		Negative	X			1 brother	1 uncle	3 aunts	2 male	3 male 3 female	0	0	0
6	X	X	Sister	Negative		2 nephews	Brother; niece	4 brothers 1 sister	3 aunts 1 uncle	1 aunt 4 uncles	'many' (25–30 at least)	'many' (30–40 at least)	4	6	0
7	X	X		Negative		2 maternal aunts	Mother; brother	1 brother	5 aunts 2 uncles	1 aunt 3 uncles	'many'	'many'	1	1	3 female
8	X	X		Negative	X	(1 sister, cousin, & nephew are schizophrenic)		2 sisters	4 aunts 6 uncles	1 aunt 5 uncles	'many'	'many'	1	3	0
9	X			2 paternal cousins (1 male; 1 female) (not 1st cousins)		Maternal male 1st cousin bipolar; Maternal aunt bipolar illness	Maternal male 1st cousin suicide	3 brothers 2 sisters	4 aunts 2 uncles	1 aunt 4 uncles	'many'	'many'	1	2	0

Appendix I—Family history data
Bipolar MS group (continued)

Subject	*Source of data* *Pt*	*Case record*	*Fam*	*Incidence MS in family*	*Incidence of affective disorder in family* *Negative*	*Bipolar illness*	*Unipolar illness*	*No. of male & female siblings*	*No. of maternal aunts & uncles*	*No. of paternal aunts & uncles*	*No. of maternal cousins male & female*	*No. of paternal cousins male & female*	*No. of nieces*	*No. of nephews*	*No. of children male & female*
10	X	X	sisters	Negative	X			1 brother 2 sisters	4 aunts 2 uncles	4 aunts 2 uncles	3 male 2 female	2 male 4 female	5	1	1 male 1 female
11	X			Negative		Maternal grandmother; 2 aunts	Maternal aunt depressed	2 brothers	unknown	unknown	unknown	unknown	unknown	unknown	2 (sex unknown)
12	X	X	daughter	Maternal female, 1st cousin			brother; maternal uncle treated for alcoholism	2 brothers 2 sisters	4 aunts 1 uncle	4 uncles	'many'	'many'	9	5	1 male 1 female
13		X		Paternal uncle		Paternal uncle treated for hypomania (same uncle has MS)	2 paternal uncles & father committed suicide	unknown	No. of unknown (at least 3 uncles)	unknown	unknown	unknown	unknown	unknown	3 (sex unknown)
14	X	X		unknown			Father alcoholic & depressed but not treated	0	unknown	unknown	unknown	unknown	unknown	unknown	unknown
15	X	X		2 paternal cousins		Brother	Maternal grandfather (psychiatric hospital-ization —alcoholism)	1 brother	unknown	unknown	unknown	unknown	unknown	unknown	unknown

Appendix I—Family history data
Unipolar MS group

Subject	*Source of data* Pt	*Case record*	*Fam*	*Incidence MS in family*	*Incidence of affective disorder in family* Negative	*Bipolar illness*	*Unipolar illness*	*No. of male & female siblings*	*No. of maternal aunts & uncles*	*No. of paternal aunts & uncles*	*No. of maternal cousins male & female*	*No. of paternal cousins male & female*	*No. of nieces*	*No. of nephews*	*No. of children male & female*
16	X	X		Negative	X			2 brothers 2 sisters	1 aunt 3 uncles	3 aunts 4 uncles	4 male 4 female	10 male 10 female	5	5	2 male
17	X	X		Negative	X			2 brothers	3 aunts 6 uncles	5 aunts 2 uncles	9 male 7 female	'many'	1	2	1 male 1 female
18	X	X		Negative		(1 maternal aunt hospitalized for psychiatric illness but diagnosis unknown)		1 brother 1 sister	4 aunts	3 aunts 1 uncle	1 male 6 female	'many'	6	2	0
19	X	X	Mother & father	Negative	X			0	1 uncle	1 uncle	2 male	1 male 1 female	0	0	0
20	X	X	Brother	Negative	X			2 brothers 3 sisters	2 aunts 4 uncles	6 aunts 1 uncle	4 male 5 female	9 male 16 female	5	3	0
21	X	X		Negative	X			1 sister	1 uncle	1 uncle	1 male 1 female	1 male	3	2	0
22	X	X		Negative	X			1 brother 2 sisters	1 aunt 1 uncle	5 aunts 1 uncle	2 male 3 female	5 male 5 female	1	3	3 male 1 female
23	X	X		Negative	X			2 brothers 2 sisters	1 aunt 1 uncle	0	5 female	0	0	0	0
24	X	X	Mother	Negative	X	(1 maternal aunt treated as outpatient for 'nervous disorder')		2 brothers 5 sisters	2 aunts 1 uncle	1 aunt 1 uncle	1 male 4 female	4 male	0	0	0
25	X	X	X	Negative	X			1 sister	2 uncles	(in Poland number unknown)	1 female	unknown	2	1	1 male 2 female

Appendix I—Family history data
Unipolar MS group (continued)

Subject	Source of data: Pt	Source of data: Case record	Source of data: Fam	Incidence MS in family	Incidence of affective disorder in family: Negative	Incidence of affective disorder in family: Bipolar illness	Incidence of affective disorder in family: Unipolar illness	No. of male & female siblings	No. of maternal aunts & uncles	No. of paternal aunts & uncles	No. of maternal cousins male & female	No. of paternal cousins male & female	No. of nieces	No. of nephews	No. of children male & female
26	X	X		Negative (Mother possibly has benign MS not worked up)	X			1 brother 1 sister	0	3 uncles	0	2 male 4 female	0	1	1 male
27	X	X		Negative		(1 female cousin had 'nervous breakdown')		1 sister	3 aunts 1 uncle	4 aunts	1 male 7 female	4 male 3 female	0	0	1 male
28	X			Negative	X			0	1 aunt 2 uncles	1 aunt 2 uncles	2 male 2 female	3 male 3 female	0	0	1 female
29	X	X		Negative	X			3 brothers	2 uncles	1 aunt 2 uncles	5 female	9 male 2 female	3	5	0
30	X	X		Negative	X			1 brother	1 aunt	1 aunt 1 uncle	1 male 2 female	4 male 3 female	0	0	0
31	X	X	Daughter	Negative			Daughter treated for depression	1 brother	unknown	2 uncles	unknown	unknown	unknown	unknown	1 male 3 female

Appendix I—Family history data
MS controls

Subject	*Source of data* Pt	*Case record*	*Fam*	*Incidence MS in family*	*Incidence of affective disorder in family* Negative	*Bipolar illness*	*Unipolar illness*	*No. of male & female siblings*	*No. of maternal aunts & uncles*	*No. of paternal aunts & uncles*	*No. of maternal cousins male & female*	*No. of paternal cousins male & female*	*No. of nieces*	*No. of nephews*	*No. of children male & female*
32	X			Paternal grand-mother definite MS & paternal aunt prob-able MS	X		(Paternal aunt alcoholism, 10–12 beers a day, never hospitalized)	1 brother 2 sisters	1 aunt 2 uncles	1 aunt	6 male 5 female	0	0	0	0
33	X			Negative	X			2 brothers	3 uncles	2 aunts	7 male 1 female	3 male 3 female	1	3	1 female
34	X			Negative	X			1 sister	2 aunts	1 aunt 3 uncles	3 male 3 female	'4 male 3 female	0	2	1 male 2 female
35			Mother	Negative	X			0	1 aunt 1 uncle	1 aunt 1 uncle	3 male	3 male 3 female	0	0	0
36	X	X		Negative	X			1 brother	4 uncles	1 aunt 2 uncles	3 male 1 female	1 male 3 female	1	1	0
37	X	X	Husband	Negative	X			1 brother 1 sister	2 aunts	3 aunts 3 uncles	6 male 1 female	3 male 5 female	1	1	1 male
38	X		Husband	Negative	X			1 half-sister	unknown	unknown	unknown	unknown	unknown	unknown	3 male 2 female
39	X			Negative		(Great uncle hospital-ized but diagnosis unknown—in state hospital for about 50 years)	Brother committed suicide	1 brother 2 sisters	1 aunt	1 aunt 1 uncle	1 male	6 male 3 female	0	0	1 male
40	X			Negative	X			1 sister	0	1 aunt 2 uncles	0	1 male 2 female	0	2	4 male
41			Wife	Negative	X			3 brothers	1 aunt 3 uncles	2 aunts 2 uncles	3 male 8 female	6 male 9 female	3	3	1 male 4 female

Appendix I—Family history data
MS controls (continued)

Subject	Source of data: Pt	Source of data: Case record	Source of data: Fam	Incidence MS in family	Incidence of affective disorder in family: Negative	Incidence of affective disorder in family: Bipolar illness	Incidence of affective disorder in family: Unipolar illness	No. of male & female siblings	No. of maternal aunts & uncles	No. of paternal aunts & uncles	No. of maternal cousins male & female	No. of paternal cousins male & female	No. of nieces	No. of nephews	No. of children male & female
42	X			Negative	X			4 brothers 1 sister	1 aunt 1 uncle	3 aunts	1 male 2 female	4 male 4 female	3	7	2 male
43	X	X		Negative	X			3 brothers 2 sisters	1 aunt 1 uncle	3 uncles	1 male 1 female	3 male 5 female	5	6	2 male 3 female
44	X	X	Husband	Negative	X			0	2 aunts	1 aunt	1 male 1 female	2 male	0	0	1 male 2 female

Appendix II

Multiple sclerosis—Bipolar group

Sex	*Subject Am. J. Psychiatr.*[†] *86*	*HLA Lab. No.*	*Family history of affective disorder*	*HLA-A*	*HLA-C*	*HLA-B*	*w4/w6*	*HLA-DR*	*w52/w53*	*HLA-DQ*	
Female	1	MD003	Positive	2,11	w4	7,35	w6	w6	w52	w1	
Female	2	MD001	Positive	1,3	w4	8,35	w6	3,w8	w52	**	
Male	3	MD005	Negative	1,24	w3	8,w62	w6	3,5	w52	w3	
Female	4	MD009	Positive	1,32		8,w61	w6	3,5	w52	w3	
Female	5	MD008	Negative	1,3	w4	35,w52	w4,w6	2		w1	
Female	7	MD010	Positive	3,24	w2,w6	35,w47	w4,w6	2,7	w53	w1	
Female	8	MD011	Positive	1,11	w4	8,35	w6	3,w6	w52	w1	No test
Female	9	MD020	Negative	3,29		7,14	w6	2		w1	for DQw2
Female	10	MD021	Positive	3,28	w3	18,w62	w6	5	w52	w3	
Female		MD026	Negative	2,24	w3,w4	35,w62	w6	4*	w53	w1	
Female		MD025	Positive	2,26	w6	7,45	w6	2,7	w53	w1,w2	
Female		MD035	Negative	1,2	w6	17,45	w4,w6	2,5	w52	w1	
Male		MD030	Positive	3,11	w3	7,w22	w6	2		w1	
Male		MD031	Negative	1,23	w4	7,44	w4,w6	3*	w52	w2,w3	
Female		MD032	Positive	3,24	w1	7,51	w4,w6	2,5	w52	w1,w3	

Multiple sclerosis—Unipolar group

Subject		*Family history of affective disorder*								
Sex	*HLA Lab. No.*		*HLA-A*	*HLA-C*	*HLA-B*	*w4/w6*	*HLA-DR*	*w52/w53*	*HLA-DQ*	
Female	MD002	Negative	2,31	w4	7,35	w6	2,5	w52	w1,w3	} No test for DQw2
Female	MD016	Negative	1,28	w4	w53,w58	w4	7	**	**	
Female	MD012	Positive	1,11	w4	8,35	w6	7*	w53	w1	
Female	MD006	Negative	2,28	w6	14,35	w6	1*	w52	w1,w3	
Female	MD004	Negative	2,23	w5	44	w4,w6	4,w8	w52,w53	w3	
Female	MD013	Negative	1,11	w4	8,35	w6	1,3	w52	w1	
Male	MD015	Negative	1,24	w4	35,w57	w4,w6	1,2		w1	
Female	MD018	Negative	2,24	w1,w2	27,w62	w4,w6	1,4	w53	w1,w3	
Female	MD019	Negative	2,24	w2	7,27	w4,w6	1,4	w53	w1,w3	
Female	MD024	Negative	1,30	w6	8,13	w4,w6	3,w6	w52	w1,w2	
Female	MD023	Negative	1,2	w3	8,w62	w6	3,4	w52,w53	w2,w3	
Female	MD027	Negative	2,26	w2	7,44	w4,w6	2		w1	
Female	MD028	Negative	1,3	w2	8,27	w4,w6	2		w1	
Female	MD033	Negative	3,32	w3	8,w60	w6	3,5	w52	w2,w3	
Female	MD036	Negative	1,23		8,w41	w6	2,4	w53	w1,w2	
Female	MD037	Positive	1,30	w4	w53	w4	w6	w52	w1	

Affective status uncertain

Sex	*Subject* *HLA Lab. No.*	*Family history of affective disorder*	*HLA-A*	*HLA-C*	*HLA-B*	*w4/w6*	*HLA-DR*	*w52/w53*	*HLA-DQ*	
Male	MS002	Unknown	2,24	w3	44,w62	w4,w6	3,4	w52,w53	w3	
Male	MS007	Unknown	2,26	w1,w2	7,27	w4,w6	2		w1	
Female	MS010	Unknown	2,32	w4	35,44	w4,w6	2,3	w52	w1	
Female	MS012	Unknown	3,25	w2	8,27	w4,w6	3,w6	w52	w1	
Male	MS013	Unknown	3,11		7,18	w6	2,4	w53	w1,w3	
Female	MS014	Unknown	3,24	w1	w22,w63	w4,w6	w6,w8	w52	w1,w3	No test for DQw2
Male	MS015	Unknown	1,3		7,17	w4,w6	2,w6	w52	w1	
Female	MS019	Unknown	2,29	w3	w41,w60	w6	w6,w9	w52,w53	w1,w3	
Male	MS020	Unknown	24,w36	w2	18,51	w4,w6	2,w6	w52	w1	
Female	MS021	Unknown	2,3		7	w6	2		w1	
Female	MS023	Unknown	2	w3,w6	w22,w57	w4,w6	2,4	w53	w1,w3	
Male	MD038	Unknown	24,30	w3	13,w62	w4,w6	4,7	w53	w2,w3	

No affective disorder group

Subject		Family history of affective disorder								
Sex	*HLA Lab. No.*		*HLA-A*	*HLA-C*	*HLA-B*	*w4/w6*	*HLA-DR*	*w52/w53*	*HLA-DQ*	
Female	MD017	Negative	24,30		w63	w4	3,w6	w52	w1,w2	
Male	MD014	Negative	2,3	w2	7,27	w4,w6	2,4	**	**	
Male	MD022	Negative	2,3		14,51	w4,w6	1*	w52	w1	
Male	MD029	Negative	3,32	w3	8,w60	w6	3,5	w52	w2,w3	
Female	MD034	Negative	1,2	w2	44,49	w4	1,w6	w52	w1	
Female	MD039	Negative	3,w34	w1	14,27	w4,w6	2,4	w53	w1,w3	
Female	MD040	Negative	1,29	w7	8,44	w4,w6	3*	w52	w2,w3	
Female	MS022	Positive	2,28		7,18	w6	2,4	w53	w1,w3	No test for DQw2
Female	MS016	Negative	2,3		14,44	w4,w6	4,w6	w52,w53	w1,w3	No test for DQw2
Male	MS017	Negative	2,24	w3	7,w62	w6	2,4	w53	w1,w3	No test for DQw2
Male	MS011	Negative	2		8,37	w4,w6	3,w6	w52	w1	No test for DQw2
Male	MS018	Negative	3,24	w4	35	w6	1,w6	w52	w1	No test for DQw2
Female	MS008	Negative	2,24		7,44	w4,w6	2,7	**	**	No test for DQw2

*Probably heterozygous for DRX based on w52, w53, or DQ type.
**Not typed.
†These patients reported in Schiffer, R. B., Wineman, N. M. & Weitkamp, L. R. Association between bipolar affective disorders and multiple sclerosis. *Am. J. Psychiatr.* 1986; **143**, 94–95.

VIII

PROPHYLACTIC APPROACH

19

WHEN SHOULD THE PATIENT WITH MULTIPLE SCLEROSIS BE TOLD HIS DIAGNOSIS?

Egon Stenager, Lone Knudsen and Knud Jensen

Clinical Neuropsychiatric Research Unit, Departments of Neurology, Clinical Psychology and Psychiatry, Odense University Hospital, Odense, Denmark

Summary

Of 46 patients with definite MS, 43 were aware of their diagnosis. Of the 43 patients, 41 wanted to be involved in the diagnostic process from the onset of MS. Those not informed at the time of diagnosis expressed dissatisfaction. Those informed at the time of diagnosis were pleased.

Introduction

This article concerns advice and guidance which can be vital when helping the patient with multiple sclerosis (MS) to attain the best possible quality of life. To achieve this it is essential that circumstances tending to exacerbate the disease are clearly explained to the patient; in other words a prophylactic attitude to the disease and its treatment must be adopted. It is thought-provoking that so few studies deal with this aspect, especially since the questions most likely to be posed by the patient are 'what worsens my condition?' and 'how can I prevent it from becoming worse?'

The leading question for the neurologist, however, is 'when should the patient be told the diagnosis?' Neurologists are very familiar with this question but many hesitate in telling the patient the diagnosis, partly because it is difficult to establish with certainty and partly because it is difficult to predict the individual prognosis. There may also be anxiety about the patient's reaction on being presented with the diagnosis, with the possibility that there might be a violent reaction, perhaps even suicide. In addition, for many MS patients the course may be mild physically, and the neurologist may perhaps feel that the patient should not be burdened with a diagnosis which, in the eyes of many laymen, is tantamount to life in a wheelchair. How does the patient experience this situation? Burnfield *et al.*,[1-3] on the basis of their own experience when advising patients, describe the difficulties that arise in connection with acknowledgement of the disease and when the patient is insufficiently informed of its consequences. Only one systematic investigation has been undertaken, namely that by Elian & Dean.[4] They made an assessment of how widespread was the wish to know the diagnosis. In a series of 167 patients they found that 83 percent wanted to know the diagnosis, 13 percent were indifferent, 4 percent did not want to know, and about one quarter did not know their diagnosis. In this chapter, the results of a small interview investigation of MS patients are presented. Two aspects were examined: (1) when, according to the patient, should the diagnosis be made known to him? and (2) how did the patient learn of the diagnosis?

Method

The first 46 patients who entered the investigation already described in this volume (chapters 4 and 16) were interviewed. They were divided into two age groups (Table 1). The patients had had their first admission within the period 1.4.1973—31.12.1985. Professional attitudes towards information as experienced by the patient ranged from reticence as long as the diagnosis was not definite, to openness from the time of the first admission if the patient appeared interested.

The following information was recorded for the patients who were aware of their diagnosis: (1) The time when they were informed; (2) the mode of learning about the diagnosis; (3) whether or not they were satisfied with the way in which it became known to them; (4) the point in the course of the disease at which they felt patients should be informed of the diagnosis.

Using this information it was possible to classify the patients into two groups as follows: (1) patients who were informed during first admission; and (2) patients who learned of their diagnosis at a later stage—during a later admission, from their general practitioner, from their spouse or by mistake.

It became obvious that the question of relevant information occupied the minds of the patients a great deal, as they themselves brought the subject up at an early stage in the interview.

The following data were also collected: scores on Kurtzke Disability Status Scale (KDSS)[5]; duration of the disease from first symptom; and duration of the disease from time of diagnosis. The diagnosic criteria used were those of Poser *et al.*[6]

Results

Table 1 shows the details of the patients included in the study. As can be seen in the Table, the age groups were 36–40 years, and 41–45 years. All had 'definite' MS. Mean values on KDSS were highest for the older group. This group has also the longest period of illness, reckoned both from time of self-reported first symptom and from time of diagnosis. The length of time from first symptom to diagnosis should be noted. As can be seen, only three were unaware of their diagnosis.

Table 2 gives details about the time when the patients were informed of their diagnosis. The upper part of the Table describes the patients who were informed of their diagnosis during their first admission. All were satisfied with this, and there was no disparity between the two age groups.

The lower part of the Table describes the patients who were told their diagnosis during a later admission or in another way. It can be seen that most were dissatisfied with this, and again there was no disparity between the two age groups.

Table 1. *Patients included in the study.*

		Age groups (years) 36–40	41–45
Sex	male	11	8
	female	14	13
Poser *et al.* criteria	CDMS A1*	22	19
	LSDMS B2†	3	2
Kurtzke Disability Status Scale	mean	3.8	4.5
	range	1–8	1–7
Duration since 1st symptom (years)	mean	10.4	17.6
	range	3–27	4–31
Duration since diagnosis (years)	mean	5.7	9.8
	range	1–13	2–31
Diagnosis	known	23	20
	unknown	2	1

*Clinical definite multiple sclerosis
†Laboratory-supported definite multiple sclerosis

Table 2. *Time of imparting diagnosis.*

Age group (years)	*Content*	*Discontent*	*Total*
(a) Patients informed of their diagnosis at the 1st neurological admission			
36–40	12	0	12
41–45	8	0	8
Total	20	0	20
(b) Patients informed of their diagnosis later than the 1st neurological admission or in other ways			
36–40	1	10	11
41–45	3	9	12
Total	4	19	23

Fisher's exact test for comparison between age groups: $P=0.27$

The patients who were informed of their diagnosis during their first admission are compared with those who learned of it at a later point in Table 3. The difference is significant. Those who were informed from the start were satisfied, and those who were not informed at that stage were dissatisfed ($p<0.005$).

Table 4 shows the responses to the question concerning when the patients would have liked to have been informed. As can be seen, only two of the 43 patients would have preferred to have been informed first when the diagnosis was certain. The others wished to have been involved in the diagnostic process from the start.

Table 3. *Comparison of patients who were informed of their diagnosis at their 1st neurological admission or in another way.*

	Content	*Discontent*	*Total*
1st admission	20	0	20
Other ways	4	19	23
Total	24	19	43

Mantel-Haenszel's test between the groups: $P<0.005$

Table 4. *Comparison between patients wishing to be informed when MS is suspected and patients wishing to be informed when a definite diagnosis of MS is being considered.*

	Age group 36–40 years	*Age group 41–45 years*	*Total*
MS suspected	23	18	41
Definite diagnosis	0	2	2
Total	23	20	43

Mantel-Haenszel's test between the groups: $P<0.005$

From Table 1, it can be seen that in the younger group almost 5 years elapsed, and in the older group almost 8, from the first symptom until the diagnosis was reached. A period of 3.2 years (range 0–7 years) passed before those patients who were not initially informed of their probable diagnosis subsequently learned of it. Further, it should be noted that 17 patients (37 percent) came to the conclusion themselves that they were suffering from MS. One of these had not had her suspicion verified at the time of the study. In five cases (11 percent) the patient's spouse alone was informed of the diagnosis. Both patient and spouse were dissatisfied with this form for procedure.

Conclusions

From these findings it is clear that when asked, almost all patients wished to be involved in the diagnostic process from the start. All the patients in our investigation have definite MS, but with a wide range of degree of physical disability. They are patients who, on average, experienced symptoms for more than 5 years before a diagnosis was reached—a period equivalent to that found by Steward & Sullivan.[7] A number of patients were forced to wait, on average, a further 3 years before being told their diagnosis, that is 8–10 years after they experienced their first symptom. It is not surprising, therefore that the great majority claim they felt relief on learning of the diagnosis, and that this relief was much more pronounced than the consternation and depression most would associate with severe disease.

As pointed out by Burnfield,[3] it is likewise understandable that these patients felt let down by their physician when they had not been informed of the nature of their disease but left to live in uncertainty for years, and to speculate on various terrible diagnostic possibilities. It seems that the truth is seldom harder to accept than the unknown, as maintained by Burnfield.[3] Both Firnhaber[8] and Burnfield[3] point out that lack of medical information can be detrimental to the doctor/patient relationship. When the patient is told the diagnosis, one should, as pointed out in an editorial in the Lancet,[9] also be prepared to follow it up and take the time necessary to describe the disease and its possible consequences for both patient and family.

On the basis of the literature on this subject and of this small study, it must be concluded that the patient should as far as possible be involved in the diagnostic process from the beginning, so that a stable basis on which a co-operative and trusting doctor/patient relationship is formed. This is also fundamental if the guidance and advice given to the patient and his family is to be of any use in the achievement of a full life with MS. It is also obvious that a good patient/doctor relationship is necessary if studies on prophylaxis are to be at all realistic.

Acknowledgements—This work was supported by Fonden for Scleroseramte på Fyn and the Danish Multiple Sclerosis Society.

References

1 Burnfield, A. & Burnfield, P. (1978): Common psychological problems in multiple sclerosis. *Br. Med. J.* **1**, 1193–1194.
2 Burnfield, A. & Burnfield, P. (1982): Psychosocial aspects of multiple sclerosis. *Physiotherapy* **68**, 149–156.
3 Burnfield, A. (1984): Doctor-patient dilemmas in multiple sclerosis. *J. Med. Ethics* **10**, 149–156.
4 Elian, M. & Dean, G. (1985): To tell or not to tell the diagnosis of multiple sclerosis. *Lancet* **i**, 27–28.
5 Kurtzke, J. F. (1983): Rating neurologic impairment in multiple sclerosis. *Neurology* **33**, 1444–1452.
6 Poser, C. M., Paty, D., Scheinberg, L. *et al.* (1983): New diagnostic criteria for multiple sclerosis: Guidelines for research protocols. *Ann. Neurol.* **13**, 227–231.
7 Stewart, D. C. & Sullivan, T. J. (1982): Illness behaviour and the sick role in chronic disease. The case of multiple sclerosis. *Soc. Sci. Med.* **16**, 1397–1404.
8 Firnhaber, W. (1986): Äufklarung bei Multiple Sklerose. *Dtsch. Med. Wochenschr.* **111**, 356.
9 Editorial (1985): Telling patients with multiple sclerosis. *Lancet* **1**, 26.

20

THE INFLUENCE OF PREGNANCY ON PHYSICAL DISABILITY AND COGNITIVE DYSFUNCTION IN MULTIPLE SCLEROSIS

Elsebeth N. Stenager, Egon Stenager, Lone Knudsen and Knud Jensen

Clinical Neuropsychiatric Research Unit, Departments of Neurology, Clinical Psychology and Psychiatry, Odense University Hospital, Odense, Denmark

Summary

For 64 female multiple sclerosis (MS) patients with early onset of the disease (15–25 years of age) and pregnancy after or during onset of MS, a risk that the pregnancy was detrimental for prognosis was indicated when the disease was assessed by the Kurtzke Disability Status Scale. On neuropsychological testing no significant differences were found, but there was a trend for women with children to perform best on the tests. MS patients did not perform as well as controls. No differences were found between the two groups for living conditions.

Introduction

What advice should be given on the question of whether or not to have children has long been a problem for the therapist involved in the care of women with multiple sclerosis.

The first extensive investigations on pregnancy and childbirth in relation to MS were carried out in the 1950s.[1] Since then, there have been several studies on how the course of this disease, assessed on physical handicaps, is influenced by pregnancy and childbirth.[2–4] The results of these investigations have on the whole been consistent. To a certain extent, pregnancy protects against relapse while childbirth increases the risk of deterioration, both in the puerperium and for at least 6 months after delivery.

No reliable evidence that pregnancy and childbirth worsen the long-term prognosis for the disease has been found. So far, only a single investigation[4] has included data on age at onset of the disease, disease duration and age at the time of the investigation in the assessment of results. In that investigation, the results were consistent with those found hitherto. Furthermore, no earlier investigation has examined how the cognitive deficits seen in MS patients are affected by pregnancy or childbirth, nor has an assessment been made of the effect on the cognitive deficits of a life at home with children and the demands this makes on the patient.

This chapter reports two investigations. The purpose of the first was to establish whether pregnancy and childbirth in the long run aggravate the physical handicaps of the MS patient, and whether, in the short term, they can cause a deterioration in the patient's condition in the postnatal period. For this we used the Kurtzke Disability Status Scale (KDSS).[5] The aim of the second investigation was to clarify the extent to which cognitive deficits are affected by pregnancy and childbirth and in addition to reveal any differences there might be in civil status between female MS patients and women in the general population in Denmark.

On the basis of the investigation, an attempt has been made to compile guidelines that could be useful when advising female patients on the question of having children. In this connection, it must be emphasized that it is absolutely essential that the patient in question is fully informed about the possible consequences of the disease at the time the diagnosis is made, so that the question of children can be realistically discussed at any stage of the disease by the patient and the therapist. In this way it should be possible to gain insight into the situation and help the patient and her partner to realise the scope of their potential and the resources they possess for coping with a child.

Materials and methods

Each investigation involved 64 patients. Because of disparity in inclusion criteria between the investigations, a few cases are included in one but not in the other study and *vice versa*. In both investigations the patients are classified into three groups as follows:

Group 1. Women with no children.

Group 2. Women with disease onset after the last pregnancy.

Group 3. Women whose disease onset was before or concomitant with pregnancy or childbirth.

In the first investigation[6] the following data were recorded for every case in each group: age at onset, age at the time of investigation, duration of the disease, scores on KDSS, number of births, whether or not there was exacerbation of MS in conjunction with pregnancy or childbirth, and number of children.

The classification procedure was the same in the second investigation as in the first. In addition, a control group of healthy persons was compiled for whom a neuropsychological assessment was made. The control group contained 18 women who were matched with those in the investigation groups for age and social class.[7] The following data were recorded for each group: age at time of study, scores on KDSS, number of children, number of children living at home, and the patient's marital status.

The following neuropsychological tests were carried out[8-13]:

WAIS-R subtest scale: scores for information, vocabulary and similarities.

Memory tests: Auditive Verbal Learning Test with delayed recall; Story Recall; Recurring Figures.

Test for attention and perceptual motor speed: Trail making test—part A and B. The Symbol Digit Modalities Test with written administration.

Results

The results of the first investigation are shown in Table 1. It can be seen that women in group 3 (disease onset prior to or in conjunction with pregnancy or childbirth) were the

Table 1. *Composition of groups in the first investigation (see text).*

	Group 1	*Group 2*	*Group 3*
No. of patients	13	28	23
Age at onset (years)	30.6	32.5	24.0
Age at examination (years)	42.6	44.1	39.8
Duration of disease (years)	11.7	12.7	16.4
KDSS score*	3.5	3.7	4.8
No. of completed pregnancies	0	61	53
Deterioration	0	0	13
Onset of disease	0	0	14
No. of children (mean, per patient)	0	2.2	2.3

*KDSS: Kurtzke Disability Status Scale.

youngest at the time of disease onset, their disease duration was longest and their scores on KDSS were the highest.

When the results are standardized for age at onset, disease duration and age at the time of study, it is found that the women in group 3 are at greater risk of long-term deterioration than those in groups 1 and 2 (multiple regression analysis F-test $P<0.05$). This finding is not consistent with those of earlier investigations.

We found that pregnancy and childbirth aggravated the disease, a finding consistent with those in other investigations. It should be noted that in contrast to several other investigations, the present one includes only a few women who had an abortion (three out of 117 pregnancies).

Table 2 shows the composition of the groups in the second investigation. The results of the Auditive Verbal Test with delayed recall are given in the Figure. For groups 1, 2 and 3 the results of the Short Term Memory and Delayed Recall tests were significantly worse than those for the control group (Student's t-test $P<0.05$). The women in all three groups therefore had some degree of learning deficit. There was a trend for women in group 1 to perform worse than those in groups 2 and 3, but the difference was not statistically significant.

The same tendency was found in all the neuropsychological tests, with women in groups 2 and 3 tending to perform better than those in group 1. It should be noted however, that group 3 contained the youngest patients—on average 39 years—who had the highest KDSS scores (mean = 4.5), and the largest number of children living at home (1.5 per patient).

As the test results could be influenced by age and KDSS,[14] paired matching was carried out for these variables in the three groups. No statistically significant differences were found,

Table 2. *Composition of groups in the second investigation (see text).*

	Group 1	*Group 2*	*Group 3*	*Control Group*
No. of patients	14	29	21	18
Age at examination (years)	41.5	45.0	39.2	41.1
KDSS score*	3.8	3.7	4.5	
No. of children	0	65	47	
No. of children living at home (mean per family)	1.0	1.5		

*KDSS: Kurtzke Disability Status Scale.

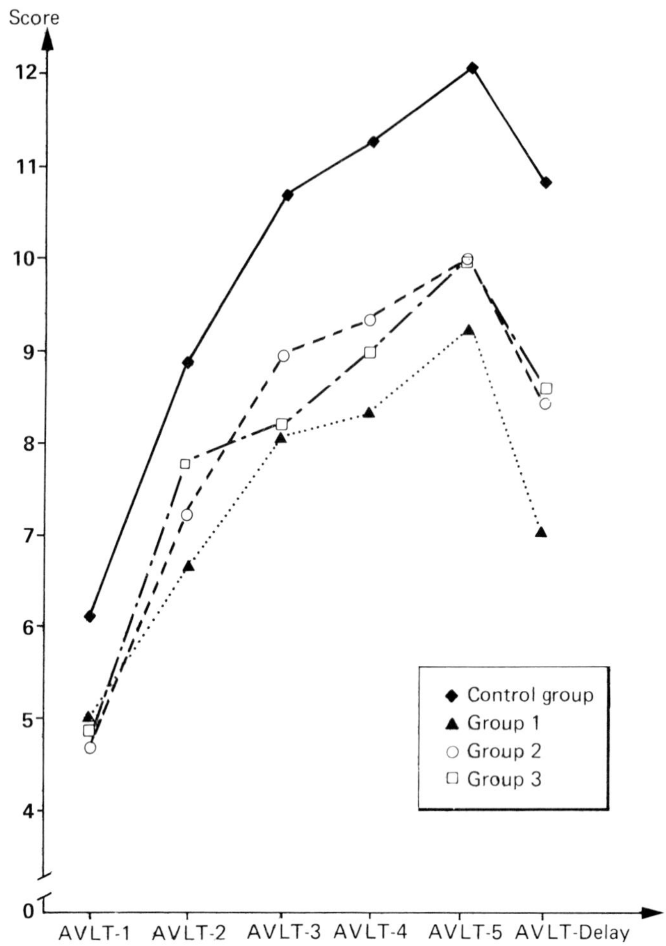

Figure. *Auditive Verbal Learning Test with delay.*

although the trend to lower scores in group 1 was repeated. Paired matching was also carried out for the following variables: age at onset, age at time of investigation, and duration of disease. No significant differences were found between the three groups, though again the trend towards better results in groups 2 and 3 than in group 1 was repeated.

Table 3 describes the family status of the MS patients. The percentage of women with the disease who lived with a spouse was equivalent to that found in the general

Table 3. *Observed and expected family status of female MS patients.*

	Observed	*Expected*
Married	43	45
Cohabiting	8	?
Divorced	3	6.7
Widows	4	1.3
Single	6	10.2

population.[15] The percentage of single or divorced women with MS was less than that found in the general population.

Discussion

In this investigation, we found that women with MS are at risk of further long-term deterioration in their condition if they have children. We found that there was risk of transient aggravation of the disease in relation to pregnancy and childbirth, and also that women with MS were no more liable to marital breakdown than women in the general population.

At the same time, the investigation of cognitive function in MS patients showed that the women who had a child after the diagnosis had been made, or who became ill in conjunction with pregnancy or childbirth, coped better with the neuropsychological tests than childless women, in spite of the fact that their disability was greater on KDSS rating. It could be argued that living in a family with children, and the consequent demands this makes on the sick person, tends to restrict cognitive decline. However, such a conclusion cannot be drawn on the basis of the present investigation alone.

Can the findings of these investigations be of any help to the therapist when advising the patient on the question of having children? Should abortion be encouraged because of the risk of exacerbation of the disease after childbirth? Should the patient be advised not to have children because of the likelihood of a worse long-term prognosis for the disease? Or should we advise women with MS to have a family because the exacerbation of the disease in pregnancy is transient and because having children perhaps reduces the risk of further cognitive decline? We believe the answer to these questions cannot be a clear cut yes or no. Before giving advice, each individual situation must be examined and the factors involved clearly defined. For example, is the disease in abeyance or is it active? Is the patient capable of coping with everyday demands, both physically and mentally? Has she the strength to care for the child, and if not, is it possible for her to obtain help? What is her co-habitant's attitude to the question and does the couple fully realize that the disease can intensify in time? What is the social and housing situation of the patient?

Only when all these factors have been carefully examined can advice for or against pregnancy be realistic. If the disease is in abeyance and the couple believe that together they are capable of taking on the responsibilities intrinsic in having a child, well knowing that its mother is handicapped, it is understandable that they may wish to go ahead even though it may not be recommendable.

These conclusions are seen purely in the light of the prospective mother and her disease. We have not taken any account of the situation for the child growing up in a family with a parent with a chronic disease that can be disabling both physically and mentally. In an American investigation in 1984, carried out by Peters & Esses,[16] a comparison was made between a group of children of 12–18 years, one of whose parents had MS, and a control group with healthy parents. The investigation showed that those with the chronically ill parent experienced less family cohesion and more family conflicts than those in the control group. Furthermore, the children with a parent with MS were less well equipped both intellectually and culturally than those in the control group. It is therefore important to talk with a couple who are considering having a child about this aspect as well, so that they are aware of the consequences and therefore better equipped to cope with the problems which may arise. We—as therapists—in making our patients aware of the problems ahead can help them choose ways in which to improve the quality of their lives.

Acknowledgements—This work was supported by Fonden for Scleroseramte på Fyn and the Danish Multiple Sclerosis Society. We wish to thank Jesper Boldsen, PhD, for assisting with the statistical analyses.

References

1 Millar, J. H. D., Allison, R. S., Cheeseman, E. A. & Merret, J. D. (1959): Pregnancy as a factor influencing relapse in disseminated sclerosis. *Brain* **82**, 417–426.
2 Poser, S. & Poser, W. (1982): Multiple sclerosis and gestation. *Neurology* **33**, 1422–7.
3 Birk, K. & Rudick, R. (1986): Pregnancy and multiple sclerosis. *Arch. Neurol.* **36**, 719–729.
4 Thompson, D. S., Nelson, L. M., Burns, A., Burks, J. S. & Franklin, G. M. (1986): The effect of pregnancy in multiple sclerosis: A retrospective study. *Neurology* **36**, 1097–1099.
5 Kurtzke, J. F. (1983): Rating neurologic impairment in multiple sclerosis. *Neurology* **33**, 1444–1452.
6 Stenager, E. N., Stenager, E. & Jensen, K.: Graviditet og dissemineret sclerose. En retrospektiv undersøgelse. *Ugeskrift for Læger* (in press).
7 Hansen, E. J. (1974): *Hvordan man indplacerer personer i socialforskningsinstituttets socialgruppe.* En revideret kodevejledning. 1st ed. Copenhagen: Socialforskningsinstituttet.
8 Wechsler, D. (1982): *WAIS-R Manual-Wechsler Adult Intelligence Scale Revised.* 1st ed. The Psychological Corporation. New York: Harcourt Brace Jovanovich.
9 Lezak, M. D. (1983): *Neuropsychological assessment.* 2nd ed. Oxford: Oxford University Press.
10 Barbizet, J. & Cany, E. (1968): Clinical and psychometrical study of a patient with memory disturbances. *J. Neurol.* **7**, 44–54.
11 Kimura, D. (1963): Right temporal lobe damage. *Arch. Neurol.* **8**, 264–271.
12 Rosenberg, S. J., Ryan, J. J. & Prifitera, A. (1984): Rey Auditive Verbal Learning Test performance of patients with and without memory impairment. *J. Clin. Psychol.* **40**, 785–787.
13 Smith, A. (1973): *Symbol Digit Modalities Test Manual*, 1st ed. Los Angeles: Western Psychological Services.
14 Van den Burg, W., van Zomeren, A. H., Minderhoud, M., Prange, A. J. A. & Meijer, N. S. A. (1987): Cognitive impairment in patients with multiple sclerosis and mild physical disability. *Arch. Neurol.* **44**, 494–501.
15 *Statistisl Årbog.* (1985): Copenhagen: Danmarks Statistik.
16 Peters, L. C. & Esses, L. M. (1985): Family environment as perceived by children with chronically ill parent. *J. Chron. Dis.* **38**, 301–308.

21

THE IMPORTANCE OF OCCUPATIONAL REHABILITATION FOR THE PATIENT WITH MULTIPLE SCLEROSIS

Egon Stenager, Lone Knudsen, and Knud Jensen

Clinical Neuropsychiatric Research Unit, Departments of Neurology, Clinical Psychology and Psychiatry, Odense University Hospital, Odense, Denmark

Summary

Of 115 MS patients, 24 were working. They are compared with 22 unemployed MS patients, matched for sex, age, socioeconomic status and Kurtzke disability status scale. No differences were found on cognitive functioning. Patients working had significantly lower scores on the Beck Depression Status Scale than the controls.

Introduction

The course of multiple sclerosis (MS) varies from person to person. For most patients it means 30 years or more of life with the disease.[1] The physical disability, though, is often not as great as anticipated when the diagnosis was pronounced. In an American investigation it was found that two out of three patients were still ambulant after 25 years.[2] Some patients who have had the disease for a long time may feel as though they had been ill in the past, but then, when no new symptoms or significant deterioration occurs over many years, they may consider themselves to be healthy even though they are aware of the imprint of the disease.

In Denmark a patient whose diagnosis is definite could certainly be granted a disability pension. Some of these patients feel they have been pressed into relinquishing their work and accepting the pension. This is also the case in other societies[3] and when it happens, the patient is left with many years ahead without the prospect of ever resuming work.[4] Naturally this applies particularly to patients whose work requires physical effort, while persons with a higher education, or who have been engaged in administration or office work, find it easier to retain their jobs.[5] In public debate in Denmark and in the literature,[3] patients have been described who, after a disease period, feel strong and wish to start working again, but have great difficulty in obtaining occupational rehabilitation.

Those who do find work again have often done so purely through their own unrelenting efforts, and in spite of the medical advice given them. We have therefore examined the question of a possible correlation between the patient's work situation and his wellbeing.

Materials and Methods

Our intention in this study was to see whether the patients with work were in any way dissimilar to a group of matched MS patients who were unemployed. Twenty-four of a total of 115 patients with definite MS had work. A number of these had been offered a pension but through their own initiative had remained employed, some in sheltered occupations. Such sheltered positions are to be found both in private and public undertakings. From the 95 remaining patients who were unemployed, a control group was formed of 22 persons who were matched as closely as possible for sex, age, social status and physical disability.

All patients were rated on the Kurtzke Disability Status Scale (KDSS)[6] and the Beck Depression Inventory.[7] A neuropsychological examination was carried out. The results were compared in the two groups of patients.

Results

The 24 patients who had work and the 22 unemployed control patients are compared in Table 1. It should be noted that the patients who worked covered a wide range of social

Table 1. *MS patients in work compared to MS patients out of work.*

		MS patients in work				*MS patients out of work*			
		n	*percent*	*mean*	*SD*	*n*	*percent*	*mean*	*SD*
	Male	16	66.7			14	66.6		
	Female	8	33.3			8	36.4		
	Age			42.79	8.21			42.50	9.25
	I	1	4.2						
Social	II	2	8.3			2	9.1		
status	III	5	20.8			5	22.7		
groups	IV	12	50.0			11	50.0		
	V	4	16.7			4	18.2		
				3.67	1.01			3.77	0.87
	1	5	20.8			4	18.2		
Kurtzke	2	7	29.2			3	13.6		
Disability	3	6	25.0			9	40.9		
Status	4	4	16.7			3	13.6		
Scale	5								
	6	1	4.2			2	9.1		
	7	1	4.2			1	4.5		
				2.75	1.54			2.82	1.44

Table 2. *WAIS-R subtests scores: patients in work compared to patients out of work.* Statistical comparison using Student's t-test.

		Information	Digit Span	Vocabulary	Arithmetic	Picture Arrangement	Block Design	Similarities
In work	$\bar{x}$	10.54	7.54	10.58	10.38	9.29	9.91	10.54
	SD	2.60	2.21	2.26	2.42	2.40	2.52	2.19
	n	24	24	24	24	24	24	24
Out of work	$\bar{x}$	10.32	8.00	10.64	10.45	9.86	10.45	10.27
	SD	2.61	2.13	2.38	2.65	3.73	2.56	2.47
	n	22	22	22	22	22	22	22
	P	<0.80	<0.80	<0.95	<0.95	<0.60	<0.50	<0.70

Table 3. *Memory test scores: patients in work compared to those out of work.*

		AVLT-1	AVLT-2	AVLT-3	AVLT-4	AVLT-5	AVLT delay	Story Recall	Recurring Figures Test	Visual Gestalt Test		
										Immediate	learning	delay
In work	$\bar{x}$	4.58	7.42	8.50	9.46	10.46	8.33	7.38	32.79	3.54	4.25	5.04
	SD	1.18	1.38	2.36	2.17	2.46	3.14	2.16	12.32	2.70	3.19	3.64
	n	24	24	24	24	24	24	24	24	24	24	24
Out of work	$\bar{x}$	4.64	7.09	8.36	9.14	9.95	8.18	7.55	31.23	3.38	3.80	4.52
	SD	1.73	1.93	2.01	2.78	2.94	3.26	2.77	10.65	3.23	4.34	4.02
	n	22	22	22	22	22	22	22	22	21	21	21
	P	<0.99*	<0.60*	<0.90*	<0.70*	<0.60*	<0.90*	NS†	NS†	NS†	NS†	NS†

*Student's t-test; †Mann-Whitney test; NS = not significant
AVLT = Auditive Verbal Learning Test

status scores and KDSS ratings. It might be expected that level in cognitive functioning would be a decisive factor in retaining work, so a comparison of this variable was also made.

In Table 2 WAIS-R subtests are compared. There were no significant differences between the two groups. The mean values for each group were very close, and the group having the highest mean value varied from test to test. In Table 3, the results of the memory tests are compared. Again no significant difference was found, and the mean values were almost equal. Table 4 shows the results of the tests for attention and perceptual motor speed. Here again, mean values were very close and no significant differences were found.

Thus no disparity was found between MS patients with work and others who did not work when using the following procedures: (1) strict matching for education and social position measured by social status ratings and physical disability by KDSS; (2) evaluation of cognitive functioning using intelligence tests, memory tests and attention and perceptual motor speed tests. Therefore it was not cognitive functioning that was decisive in retaining work.

We now turn to examination of variation in mental wellbeing. For this we have used Beck Depression Inventory, with which the patients self-rate possible depressive symptoms. From some of our other work (see Chapter 16) we know that there is a connection between these symptoms and KDSS. Table 5 shows that the patients in work had a significantly lower mean value ($P<0.01$) on self-rating than those who were out of work. In other words, patients who do not work had a higher frequency of symptoms.

Table 4. *Attention and Motor Perceptual Speed Test scores: patients in work compared to patients out of work.* Statistical comparisons used Mann-Whitney Test. NS = not significant.

		Trail Making part A	*Trail Making part B*	*Symbol Digit Modalities Test Written*	*Symbol Digit Modalities Test Oral*
Patients in work	$\bar{x}$	56.04	107.83	36.63	43.57
	SD	20.15	40.37	8.99	13.63
	n	24	24	24	24
Patients out of work	$\bar{x}$	56.57	106.62	36.19	42.08
	SD	20.99	42.08	10.00	9.11
	n	21	21	21	21
	P	NS	NS	NS	NS

Table 5. *Beck Depression Inventory scores: patients in work compared to those out of work.* Statistical comparison used Mann-Whitney Test.

		Beck Depression Inventory Score
Patients in work	$\bar{x}$	3.29
	SD	3.91
	n	24
Patients out of work	$\bar{x}$	7.36
	SD	5.88
	n	22

$P<0.01$

Conclusion

In two groups of MS patients who are comparable for social status, physical disability, and cognitive functioning—and thereby would seem to have the same potential for work—we have found that those *not* having work presented significantly more depressive symptoms. None of the patients in the investigation reported economic, marital or social problems. No predisposition to mental disorders was found in any of the patients and none had a history of previous mental disorder. It seems then that the precipitating factor for depressive symptoms in these patients is to be found elsewhere.

The following circumstances tended to find their expression in several depressive complaints: the experience of passivity, isolation in society, absence of stimulation that the company of colleagues and the demands of a job would bring, and feelings of uselessness—particularly when the disease is in a stable phase. All these circumstances are instrumental in making the patient's life with MS even more difficult.

Recognition of suitability for occupational rehabilitation is vital from the start of the disease. As can be seen in Table 1, there is greater intravariation in KDSS scores and social status among the group of patients with work. This means that even patients with severe disabilities can remain at work, so long as allowances are made for the disability. This does not mean that all MS patients should preferably continue to work. However, occupational rehabilitation should be considered with great care and carried out with strict relevance to individual potential. The individual patient should be ensured a realistic chance of performing within his or her scope while allowance is made for the changes and adjustment that may be necessary along the way. This requires the interdisciplinary collaboration of therapists with extensive knowledge of and interest in the field. It is equally important to take the patients' work situation into account from the start of the disease. Although it is seldom discussed with them in the initial stage, it is certain that it is a source of great worry to them. It is vital that the decisions made in the early stages and the revisions made along the way are realistic. The majority of these patients have to live with the consequences of these decisions for 30 years or more—so the decisions taken on the future of the patient are crucial for the pattern of his subsequent life.

Acknowledgements—This work was supported by Fonden for Scleroseramte på Fyn and the Danish Multiple Sclerosis Society.

References

1 Hyllested, K. (1961): Lethality, duration and mortality of disseminated sclerosis in Denmark. *Acta Psychiatr. Scand.* **36**, 553–564.
2 Percy, A. K., Nobrega, F. T., Okazaki, H. *et al.* (1971): Multiple sclerosis in Rochester, Minn.: A 60-year appraisal. *Arch. Neurol.* **25**, 105–111.
3 von Barylla, F. (1961): Zur Invalidisierung multiple Sklerosekranken unter Berüchsichtiger psychisher Veränderungen. *Zeitschrift für Psychiatrie, Neurologie und Medizinishe Psychologie.* **13**, 433–450.
4 Bauer, H. J. (1965): Prognostic criteria in multiple sclerosis. *Ann. N. Y. Acad. Sci.* **122**, 542.
5 McDonald, W. I. & Silberberg, D. H. (1986): *Multiple sclerosis*, 1st edn, p 180. London: Butterworths.
6 Kurtzke, J. F. (1983): Rating neurologic impairment in multiple sclerosis. *Neurology* **33**, 1444–1452.
7 Beck, A. T., Ward, C. H., Mendelson, M., Mock, J. & Erbaugh, J. (1961): An inventory for measuring depression. *Arch. Gen. Psychiatry* **4**, 561–571.

22

FINAL COMMENTS

Knud Jensen, Egon Stenager and Lone Knudsen

Clinical Neuropsychiatric Research Unit, Departments of Psychiatry, Neurology, and Clinical Psychology, Odense University Hospital, Odense, Denmark

Until 1838 when Carswell compiled his patho-anatomical description of the disease entity now known as multiple sclerosis (MS) and his French colleague, Cruveillier, related clinical symptoms to patho-anatomical findings, only sparse information on mental disorders was to be found in the early literature. It was, however, known that such disorders occurred and Charcot's lecture notes from 1872 clearly describe the psyche of the MS patient. Only in the last 40–60 years have more systematic studies on the mental disorders associated with multiple sclerosis been undertaken. Unfortunately, these studies have often given rise to confusion because of the lack of conformity in the methods used to describe the disorders. Therefore comparison is difficult and sometimes even impossible.

Even though mental disorders are to be expected in conjunction with a disease causing widespread lesions throughout the central nervous system, interest in such disorders or in cognitive deficits has been limited. However, in recent years some progress has been made in this direction and some research centres now carry out more systematic studies.

Knowledge is slowly progressing and the present stage of development is quite well covered in this book. Mahler *et al.* describe a screening procedure for cognitive impairment. They stress the fact that the lesions in MS have their primary site in the subcortical white matter and especially in the periventricular regions. They find that the subcortical pattern in patients with cognitive impairment is very similar to that seen in the AIDS-dementia complex, Binswanger dementia and in other diseases of the white matter. His conclusions are confirmed by Grant *et al.*, Stenager *et al.* and Fischer who, using varying methods, all found that cognitive deficits are a usual trend in the course of MS. They appear in the early stages of the disease and increase with physical disability. Magnetic resonance (NMR) scanning provides an important additional tool in the neurological clinic. As described by Paty, this sensitive method makes it possible to demonstrate the dissemination of the disease and opens the way for detection of the degree of disease activity. Callanan, Logsdail, Ron and Warrington conclude in their study that detected cognitive impairment is a very reliable indicator of brain pathology compared to conventional neurological symptoms and signs. NMR scanning shows that deficient overall ability is associated with the presence of a large number of lesions.

Rao *et al.* correlated cognitive deficits with the results of NMR scanning and they clearly describe the strong relationship found between the severity of cerebral pathology and cognitive dysfunction. It is even possible to relate NMR results to specific findings in neuropsychological investigations. Thus, they found NMR variables related to language and visuospatial scales, and mention the special significance of corpus callosum atrophy, which might explain impairment of sustained attention and rapid problem solving in cases where precisely timed interhemispheric communication is found to be disrupted. They also suggest other focal morphological structures which might be involved in some cases, producing more specific cognitive deficits. Nielsen *et al.* describe the cerebral blood flow relative to cognitive functioning in MS. They found that the cerebral blood flow decrement is secondary to cognitive deficiency.

Most studies mention methodological problems, consistency in which is essential if results are to be comparable. In this connection Knudsen *et al.* discuss the impact of specific primary visual defects on neuropsychological test results.

But can mental disorders always be explained by the MS lesions in the central nervous system? In their study, Grant *et al.* found that stressful life circumstances in the months preceding exacerbation of the disease might explain the timing of symptom exacerbation and suggest that such stressors might perturb an already unstable neuro-immunological system. Most clinicians contend that MS patients are often euphoric. However Rabins states in his study that euphoria is seldom seen, but when seen occurs predominantly in cases of very severe brain damage. Joffe, Lippert, Gray, Sawa and Horvath put forward the possibility that a structural or neurochemical brain lesion in MS may explain mood disorders and, in agreement with Minden *et al.*, call for more research on the possible mechanism of an association between MS and depression. It was found in the study of Minden *et al.* that major depressions are often preceded by exacerbations of the disease and treatment with ACTH and prednisone.

Jouvent *et al.* compared mental disorders and cognitive impairment and they found that in early MS and recent isolated optic neuritis nearly half of their patients suffered from cognitive impairment and that cognitive impairment is very frequent in MS, although patients do not complain of its effect on daily living. Stenager *et al.* concluded that when MS patients complain of depression, it can be an indication of severe progression of brain damage.

Logsdail, Callanan and Ron studied psychiatric morbidity in 76 patients with clinically isolated lesions, such as optic neuritis, and brain stem and spinal cord lesions. They did not find a significant association between the presence of NMR scanning abnormalities and psychiatric morbidity.

Schiffer *et al.* related MS to affective disorders and tried to find common genetic variables by studying family histories, sex and HLA-DR characteristics. They found a relationship and stressed the importance of psychiatric evaluation of MS patients.

In the final chapters Stenager *et al.* discusses some everyday aspects of problems connected with a chronic disease such as MS. When should the diagnosis be told to the patient? What is the influence of pregnancy on the disease? These problems are evident but often overlooked when MS and its effects on everyday living are discussed in symposia and congresses. Finally, Stenager *et al.* discuss the importance of occupational rehabilitation.

We learned a lot at the symposium about mental disorders and cognitive deficits in MS. A clear picture was gained of the present stage of development as presented by specialists representing research centres in many parts of the world. But it is obvious that there are still unsolved problems. Many of the conclusions put forward need further verification and it is clear that the extensive data now available require further processing if the individual patient is to benefit.

Greater equivalence in neuropsychological methodology is necessary before comparisons can be valid, and further reliable indicators of the severity of cognitive impairment are needed. In addition more explicit information on the depressive symptoms seen in MS is required—are the depressions seen with MS reactive, or are they part of a bipolar/unipolar manic depressive disorder? How are they related to decline in cognitive functioning? How does a physical handicap and concurrent cognitive impairment influence social life with family and friends? How can one compensate? How does the cognitive impairment influence sexuality? Will others confirm that life events and reactive depression can provoke exacerbation of the disease by disturbing an already unstable neuro-immunological system? This book does not provide the answer to all questions. It is obvious that intensive investigation adhering to epidemiological selection criteria and using standard comparable neuropsychological tests should be our aim in the future.

KEYWORD INDEX